COMPREHENSIVE TRIAGE

A Manual for
Developing and Implementing
A Nursing Care System

COMPREHENSIVE TRIAGE
A Manual for
Developing and Implementing
A Nursing Care System

June D. Thompson and Joyce E. Dains

Reston Publishing Company, Inc.
A Prentice-Hall Company
Reston, Virginia

Library of Congress Cataloging in Publication Data

Thompson, June D., 1946–
   Comprehensive triage.

   1. Emergency nursing. 2. Triage (Medicine).
3. Hospitals—Emergency service. I. Dains,
Joyce. II. Title. [DNLM: 1. Emergency
medical services—Nursing texts. 2. Nursing
care. WY 150 T473c]
RT120.E4T48   362.1′8   81-15861
ISBN 0-8359-0906-9   AACR2

© 1982 by Reston Publishing Company, Inc.
   A Prentice-Hall Company
   Reston, Virginia 22090

10   9   8   7   6   5   4   3   2   1

Printed in the United States of America

*This text was developed in concept
at the Childrens Hospital in Columbus, Ohio.*

*It is therefore dedicated
to the children everywhere
who require emergency care,
and to the health care
professionals who deliver
those services.*

June D. Thompson
Joyce E. Dains

Contents

Introduction

The word *triage* is derived from the French *trier*, meaning "to sort out." Originally, the term referred to the disposition of the injured during disasters and military situations. Today, however, the term is more commonly used to refer to the sorting of clients coming to emergency departments.

Most emergency departments have been required to initiate some type of triage system. The continued surge of emergency department utilization in this country has forced emergency department personnel to devise some method of sorting clients accessing their system. Most of the sorting systems were needed yesterday and initiated today; and many have been put into operation with little thought and few, if any, guidelines. Health care experts agree that the triage system should be the pulse of the entire emergency center's operations. Yet few triage systems are developed with adequate operational guidelines for, or adequate education of, the people who will implement the triage system.

The purpose of this book is to move step-by-step through a triage implementation process. Current system assessment; operational guidelines to initiate, maintain, and evaluate a triage system; and the education of personnel will be discussed in detail. By the time you have completed this text, you should know how to implement a triage system in your hospital.

It is our philosophy that client care begins as the client enters the emergency department doors and that the professional nurse should initially assess each client. A comprehensive triage system as described in this text enhances the initial client assessment and care provided, and incorporates periodic continued reassessment until the client is seen by the designated health care provider.

The triage process as described herein attempts to move a

significant portion of professional nursing care "into the lobby." Triage as further developed in this book consists of five major components:

1. Collection of subjective and objective data relevant to the reason the client accessed the emergency department.
2. Collection of selected information about the client's current health care practices, current health care providers, knowledge regarding the current complaint, and factors that may affect the recovery period once released from the emergency department.
3. Initiation of appropriate first aid techniques.
4. Appropriate categorization of the client which would indicate where the client will be seen, by whom, and when.
5. A schedule for periodic reassessment by triage personnel until the client is actually seen by the physician.

Triage should be far more than just the initial sorting of clients. An effective triage system provides the opportunity to accept individuals into the health care system, quickly assess that individual's needs, and make appropriate referrals. This triage system pauses for a moment to get to know each and every client. The young mother, for example, returning to the emergency department for the third time because of her "nerves" does not really need the emergency department. An astute triage nurse and an effective triage system should screen this client and make the appropriate referrals which may, in fact, divert her away from the emergency department. In contrast, the teenager who is reluctantly dragged into the emergency department because "he took some pills" would be quickly and efficiently triaged for prompt medical attention. In essence, the purpose of a complete and effective triage system is to have the individual seen by the right person, in the right place, for the right problem, at the right time.

An effective triage system will improve client flow and expedite emergency department care. The triage nurse is the first person to assess each client entering the system and it is essentially that nurse who sets the pace for the entire center's operation. Triage nursing is a most difficult and challenging position. Done well, triage is the key to an efficient department; good community relations; and, ultimately, excellent client care.

Conceptual Development of the Triage System

Part 1

Conceptual Framework

Chapter 1

The success of implementing an effective triage system is directly proportional to the institution's desire to have a triage system, the program planner's knowledge of change theory, and the ability to implement those change theory concepts in a highly complex organizational structure. Knowing what a triage system is and actually implementing a successful ongoing program are two very different processes. Many triage systems have been initiated and then have failed. Many systems currently operating are ineffective or pseudo "old" type sorting systems, which do not effectively provide accurate initial sorting or ongoing continued evaluation of clients.

The purpose of this chapter is to provide a framework for the planning and the implementation of a comprehensive triage system.

THEORETICAL FOUNDATIONS

Implementing an effective triage system in the complex organizational structure of the hospital is a difficult task. The change agent needs a framework from which to assess the system and some type of guidelines by which to implement the triage plan. The two theories that provide the best framework for planning and implementation are *planned change theory* and *systems analysis theory*. Each will be discussed briefly. The actual details of the triage plan and implementation guidelines will be presented in light of these interdependent theories.

PLANNED CHANGE

Planned change is a conscious deliberate attempt to apply new knowledge in order to modify behavior or practice. Planned change involves reeducation about current ideas, values, and practices. The implementation of a comprehensive triage system is a conscious and deliberate process. The program planner must have a plan in mind, must ready the system for the plan, and must implement the plan according to a predetermined strategy.

Kurt Lewin and Edgar Schein present the process of planned change from a practical framework of unfreezing, changing or moving, and refreezing the system (Bennis, 1969).

Unfreezing

Unfreezing is the process by which the system is readied for change. Unfreezing is probably the single most important step in the change process. The change agent must assist the organization or department to move from a stable, familiar system of operation into a state of dissatisfaction and disruption. By the completion of the unfreezing phase, involved personnel perceive the need for change and are excited to the extent that the actual change can be initiated.

Unfreezing is a very fragile period during which the change agent must assess system resistance and modify the change plan as collaborated. Information, education, and clarification must be provided for those who will be affected by the change. Enthusiasm must be engendered in order to make the change idea come alive and become a priority for the system's improvement.

In essence, the unfreezing period is the time when the change agent prepares the system for the change. By the time unfreezing is completed, the system is open and ready for a change in operating procedure.

Moving

Moving is the period during which the system implements the change. This is the time when formal and informal educational programs take place and structural renovation occurs. The change plan is formalized and implemented.

The moving portion of change is the most exciting. This is the time during which everyone has a job to do. Some jobs will be specific and technical and others will be educational and supportive. It is imperative, however, that overall everyone work as a team to actually implement the triage system.

Refreezing

Refreezing is the process of reestablishing the system at a *permanent* higher level of operation. Refreezing usually goes through a honeymoon phase when those within the system ignore or overlook little snags in the new program or slight dissatisfactions with the new program operations. However, if the small problems are not adequately assessed and addressed, they soon may become very disruptive to the new system operation.

The process of refreezing the system is very important and, in fact, will determine the system's ability to maintain the new level of operation. For the change agent or program planner, refreezing is the time to assess the mechanical functioning of the new system. The attitude of the involved employees, administration, and the community about the functioning of the new program must be evaluated. The program planner must implement an audit process and actually evaluate the effectiveness of the new program. The planner must be willing to make revisions as needed, and to support the unfreezing, moving, and refreezing as it relates to those revisions.

In essence, refreezing is an ongoing maintenance process. It is the continued monitoring and evaluation of the newly implemented program. Certainly after the program is initiated, there will be numerous wrinkles and problems. The freezing process involves working on those issues and reestablishing a higher level of system operation.

Figure 1-1 summarizes the change process from these three points. The system is stable and functioning at a given level. The change agent works to reeducate the personnel to a point of system dissatisfaction, thus *unfreezing* the system. The new ideas and program can then be implemented. The implementation phase is the *moving* part of the change process. After the change is implemented, the system must then be refrozen at this new higher level of

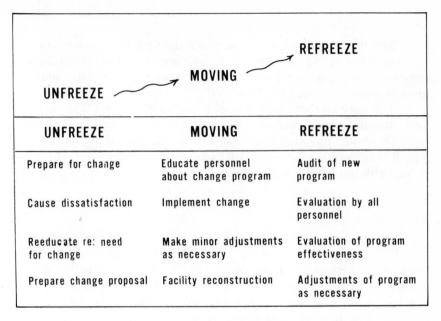

Figure 1-1   The change process.

functioning. The *refreezing* is a process of evaluation and stabilization that continues throughout the new program existence.

SYSTEMS THEORY

The framework underlying the content and commentary of this book comes from a systems perspective of triage as a concept. Triage can be analyzed systematically within the context of the complex organizational structure of a hospital.

A *system* is defined as a set of units with relationships among those units. Systems involving people that exchange matter, energy and information are called open systems. Each system has boundaries that distinguish it from other systems. The boundaries of a system determine its parameters and interface with other systems. The boundaries of a system are crucial because they determine the amount of energy and information that flows in and out of a system.

Systems are arranged in a hierarchical fashion. The organization or group that one wants to look at or work with is defined as a *target system*. Any smaller units within the target system are called *subsystems*. The next larger system outside the target system is called the *suprasystem*. The environment or the area outside the suprasystem is called the *megasystem*. The *impinging system* represents any system that operates selectively in the target system, in the suprasystem, and in the megasystem (see Figure 1-2).

TRIAGE: A SYSTEMS PERSPECTIVE

Systems theory provides an orderly method by which to analyze the triage system and those groups that interface with the triage system. Figure 1-3 portrays how the triage system is viewed within the context of systems analysis. The triage system is obviously the target system. In order to implement a triage system, one must first assess those supra-, sub-, and impinging systems that impact the triage system. These are:

1. Subsystems: triage nurse, client, ancillary support person, float nurse.
2. Impinging Systems:
    a. The physician groups working in the emergency department.

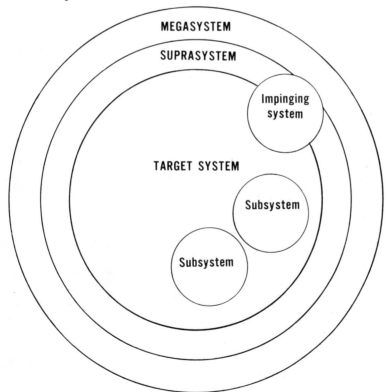

Figure 1-2   Systems concept overview.

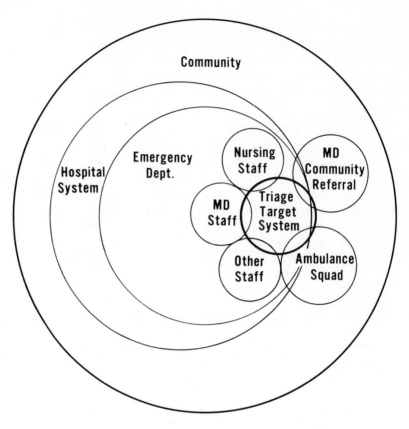

Figure 1-3   The triage system in the context of systems analysis.

  b. The nursing groups working in the emergency depart-
      ment.
  c. All other personnel working in the emergency depart-
      ment.
  d. Ambulance-squad systems bringing clients to the emer-
      gency department.
  e. Community physicians who refer clients to the emer-
      gency department.
3. Suprasystem: the emergency department in which the
   triage system functions.

4. Megasystem:
  a. The hospital representing administration and client
      services.
  b. The community that accesses the services of the hos-
      pital and the emergency department.

The process of change occurs in a variety of ways in a complex organization such as a hospital. A thorough understanding of the system components within the organization facilitates moving that system's functioning from one level of operation to another. Thus, in order to implement a comprehensive triage system, it is imperative that the change agent comprehend the system in which the change will occur and the process necessary to expedite that change.

REFERENCES

Anderson, Ralph E, and Irl Carter. Human behavior in the social environment: a social systems approach, ed. 2, New York, 1978: Aldine Publishing Company.

Bennis, Warren, Kenneth Benne, and Robert Chin. The planning of change, ed. 2., New York, 1969: Holt, Rinehart and Winston, Inc., pp. 98–107.

Bertrand, Alvin. Social organization: a general systems and role theory perspective, Philadelphia, 1972: Davis, pp. 97–105.

Overview of Triage
As a Process

Chapter 2

The concept of triage has been developed for use in three distinct settings: military, disaster, the emergency department. All these groups show similarities in needing to establish emergency care priorities. In addition each group has distinct differences in how those priorities are determined. To implement an appropriate triage system in the emergency department, it is necessary for the program planner to be familiar with the development of triage as a process.

MILITARY TRIAGE

Purpose

Triage originated on the World War I battle fields. The term was applied to the process of sorting out casualties who could be returned to the front by concentrating the limited medical resources available on their ailments. The main intent was to treat those who would then be able to return to battle. The triage technique adapted from experience in both the world wars and the Vietnam War has come to mean the process by which all injured individuals are sorted and classified according to the type and urgency of their condition. They are then transported under the assigned priorities for care.

Classification

The war-time triage classification utilizes four priority categories:

1. *Minimal care*—little or no professional treatment required. Individuals should be capable of returning to normal activities after a brief period of treatment.

2. *Immediate care*—highest priority given. This group includes those with shock, airway problems, major chest or crush injuries, partial amputation, or open fractures.

3. *Delayed care*—treatment can be postponed without loss of life, although morbidity may increase. This group includes those with simple fractures, lacerations without extensive bleeding, and non-critical injuries.

4. *Expectant care*—injuries require considerable time, effort, and supplies to treat. Individuals are expected to live even though definitive care is postponed until persons in the immediate or delayed categories are treated (Hughes, 1976).

DISASTER TRIAGE

Purpose

The concept of triage as applied to disaster or large-scale emergencies also utilizes classification categories. Priority for transportation and treatment is determined by the established categories, which facilitate the sorting process by providing parameters for decision-making. The critical feature of disaster triage is that it is field-oriented, thus all victims are not initially transported. This prevents overloading of emergency departments and allows more efficient use of available resources.

Classification

Individuals are evaluated and divided into four categories for treatment and transportation:

Class I—Emergent: individuals with critical life-threatening injuries or illnesses whose chances of survival depend upon immediate care. Examples: airway problems, hemorrhage, shock.

Class II—Urgent: victims with major injuries or illnesses who should be treated within 20 minutes to two hours and who require emergency care prior to transportation. Examples: open fractures, chest wounds.

Class III—Non-urgent: individuals with minor injuries who are usually ambulatory, or whose care can be delayed beyond two hours. Examples: closed fractures, sprains and strains.

Class IV—Dead or with impending death: victims with a slim chance of surviving who should not take priority over potentially salvageable individual. Examples: massive crushing head injury, extensive third- and fourth-degree burns.

This triage system serves to obtain maximum salvage rates with whatever medical resources are available to that particular community.

EMERGENCY DEPARTMENT TRIAGE

Purpose and Functions

Triage as performed in the emergency department differs from military and disaster triage in the scope of both purpose and function. While some clients coming to the emergency department require the same emergent screening as those victims seen in both the disaster and military triage systems, a majority of clients require a different type of prioritization schedule. A comprehensive emergency department triage system should spend minimal time prioritizing those critically ill and injured individuals needing immediate medical care. The triage system should, however, have the capacity to assess and prioritize the masses of clients with urgent and nonemergent needs.

Fourteen characteristics of a comprehensive triage system are identified. These are:

1. Expedites client care through immediate assessment by the triage person.

2. Provides the opportunity to develop a selected client data base.

3. Ensures the establishment of client care priorities according to the acuteness of the condition.

4. Decreases client delays by initiating diagnostic procedures.

5. Provides continuous reassessment of individuals waiting for treatment.

6. Provides the opportunity to identify selected client or family health-learning needs.

7. Functions as a screening area for individuals needing information.

8. Functions as a referral site for selected clients not requiring emergency care.

9. Relieves congestion in critical treatment areas and improves traffic flow through utilization of a variety of health care resources.

10. Assists in effective utilization of space and personnel through the assignment of clients to designated treatment areas.

11. Promotes rapport through immediate demonstration of concern for emergency department client problems.

12. Has built-in mechanisms for continued system evaluation.

13. Decreases anxiety levels of client and family by providing immediate and ongoing assessment while the client is waiting for medical care.

14. Improves public relations by providing initial and continued client care "in the lobby."

The types of triage systems presently used in emergency departments are discussed in Chapter 3.

Principles

There are several principles that must be applied in order to efficiently and effectively carry out triage within the emergency department:

1. The magnitude of service needs and the available resources must be known. Appropriate triage decisions will vary from situation to situation depending upon those needs and resources.

2. The triage team provides only selected first aid treatment. Further treatment would impede the triage process and significantly reduce its capabilities.

3. The triage team needs to have the capability of evaluating the client's vital signs in order to make some triage decisions.

4. The triage personnel require specialized education preparing them for functioning in the triage system.

5. Clients must be categorized according to acuteness based upon the initial assessment. This categorization will determine the prioritization for care.

6. Clients may be recategorized at any time.

7. All pertinent client data are documented in the client's emergency care record. This information is periodically updated.

8. A totally separate category of triage is necessary for radiation accidents and certain biological and chemical poison cases because of the specialized needs for decontamination.

Historical Development

Since 1940, two significant trends in emergency department utilization have been identified. The first is a marked increase in the use of emergency departments. The second is a concomitant increase in the numbers of non-urgent as well as emergent visits. These increases have been attributed to a number of medical and sociological factors:

1. The changing perception of hospitals from that of a last resort for the seriously ill to that of a 24-hour-a-day community resource where one can receive a variety of health care services.

2. The increase of physician specialization with a decrease of office-based primary care practitioners.

3. The inability or unwillingness of individuals to reach their physicians on weekends, nights, or holidays for either emergent or nonurgent appointments.

4. An increasingly mechanized, synthetic, and high-speed environment that engenders rising rates of accidental injury, toxic reactions and hypersensitivity.

5. The public's perception of the emergency department as the appropriate place for certain types of care because of sophisticated technological capabilities.

6. Higher costs of medical care coupled with health insurance that covers emergency department care but not office visits.

7. "Quick" care in the emergency department versus long waits for an office appointment.

16

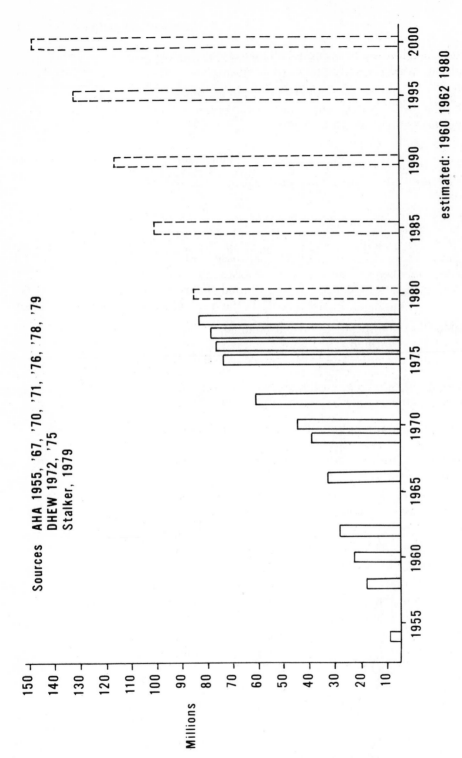

Figure 2-1 Total number of emergency department visits 1954-1980 with projections for 1985-2000.

8. The concentration of economically dependent and/or socially isolated minority groups in urban centers who lack the contacts to access the health care system in the more traditional manner.

9. An increasingly mobile population who lack primary health care providers.

10. Increasing instruction from physicians' offices for clients to use emergency care facilities when the office is closed or the physician is unavailable.

The dramatic increase in the use of emergency departments can be seen in Figure 2-1. The number of emergency department visits for the year 1954 was 9.7 million; in 1978 that figure had jumped to 83.5 million, an increase of 760 percent. This increase in client load has not been dependent upon concomitant increases in community population. The population increase in the United States for the same period is only 34 percent. Figure 2-2 shows the increase in the number of emergency department visits per 1,000 population. In 1954 there were 59.5 emergency department visits for every 1,000 persons; in 1978 that figure had increased to 382.2 visits for every 1,000 persons.

Estimates for future emergency department use can be extrapolated from least squares analysis of the data from 1954-1978. At an

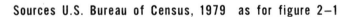

Sources U.S. Bureau of Census, 1979 as for figure 2–1

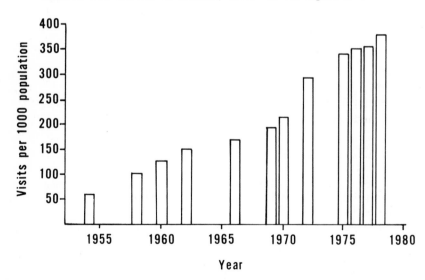

Figure 2-2 Number of emergency department visits per 1,000 population 1954-1978.

increase of 3.14 million visits per year, the number of emergency department visits will mushroom to 116 million by 1995, and 148 million by the year 2000.

Triage in hospitals emerged in the late fifties and early sixties. The development of some type of triage procedures was a direct result of the increasing volume of individuals seeking care through emergency services. The early triage systems were disorganized with the single goal of sorting out only the very emergent cases. Since the 1960s, hospitals have continued to struggle with methods to efficiently and effectively care for the consistently increasing numbers of clients.

If hospital emergency departments are to survive the projected increased department use, it is imperative that more sophisticated and comprehensive triage systems be developed. Triage as presented in this text is shown as an organized and expandable system of reception and sorting to ensure that every client receives appropriate care.

REFERENCES

American Hospital Association: Hospitals, guide issue, 29(15): part 2, August 1, 1955.

American Hospital Association: Hospitals, guide issue, 41(15): part 2, August 1, 1967.

American Hospital Association: Hospitals, guide issue, 44(15): part 2, August 1, 1970.

American Hospital Association: Hospitals, guide issue, 45(15): part 2, August 1, 1971.

American Hospital Association: Hospital statistics, 1976 ed., Chicago, 1976.

American Hospital Association: Hospital statistics, 1978 ed., Chicago, 1978.

American Hospital Association: Hospital statistics, 1979 ed., Chicago, 1979.

Erven, Lawrence W. Handbook of emergency care and rescue, revised edition, Beverly Hills, 1976: Glencoe Press.

Gazzaniga, Alan B., Lloyd T. Iseri, and Martin Baren, editors. Emergency care: principles and practices for the e.m.t.-paramedic, Reston, Va., 1979: Reston Publishing Company.

Howell, James T. and Robin C. Buerki. The emergency unit in the modern hospital, Hospitals (31):pp. 37-39 March 16, 1957.

Hughes, John H. Triage—a new look at an old concept, Postgrad. Med., 60(4):pp. 223-227, October 1976.

Lee, Sidney S., Jerry A. Solon, and Cecil G. Sheps. How new patterns of medical care affect the emergency unit, Mod. Hosp., 94(5):pp. 97-101, May 1960.

Nelson, Doris M. Triage and assessment, in Carmen G. Warner, editor: Emergency care assessment and intervention, ed. 5, St. Louis, 1978: The C.V. Mosby Co., pp. 45-57.

Nelson, Doris M. Triage in the emergency suite, Hosp. Top., 51(9):pp. 39-41. September 1973.

Nyberg, Jan. Perception of patient problems in the emergency department, J.E.N., 4(1):pp. 15-19, January/February 1978.

Shortliffe, Ernest C., T. Stewart Hamilton, and Edward H. Noroian. The emergency room and the changing pattern of medical care, N. Engl. J. Med., 258(1):pp. 20-25, January 2, 1958.

Slay, Larry E., and Wayne G. Riskin. Algorithm-directed triage in an emergency department, J.A.C.E.P., 5(11):pp. 869-876, November 1976.

Stalker, Timothy A. What's behind the explosive growth in hospital-based primary care? Hosp. Physician 15(2):pp. 26-28, February 1979.

Stratmann, William C., and Ralph Ullman. A study of consumer attitudes about health care: the role of the emergency room, Med. Care, 13(12):pp. 1033-1043, December 1975.

U.S. Bureau of the Census. Statistical abstract of the United States: 1979, ed. 100, Washington, D.C., 1979.

U.S. Department of Health, Education, and Welfare. Facts and trends on. . . hospital outpatient services, Washington, D.C., 1964, Public Health Service, Publication No. 930-C-6.

U.S. Department of Health, Education, and Welfare. Hospitals, a county and metropolitan area date book, 1972, Rockville, Md., 1975, Public Health Service, DHEW Publication No. (HRA) 75-1223.

Weinerman, E. Richard, and Herbert R. Edwards. 'Triage' system shows promise in management of emergency department load, Hospitals, 38(22):pp 55-62, November 16, 1964.

Willis, Dorothy T. A study of nursing triage, J.E.N. 5(6):pp. 8-11, November/December 1979.

Types of Emergency Department Triage Systems

Chapter 3

There are several triage systems in use that when analyzed in the context of nursing process, can be grouped into three major categories: Type 1 ("Traffic Director"), Type II ("Spot Check"), and Type III ("Comprehensive"). While all systems share the triage function of sorting clients into categories for care, the assessment, planning, implementation, and evaluation phases of the process contain areas of major difference. Table 3-1 summarizes the major differences.

TYPE I—"TRAFFIC DIRECTOR"

The major purpose of this type system is simply to differentiate those clients with emergent needs from those with non-urgent needs. Triage systems falling into this category include those considered as "basic" or "non-professional."

Table 3-1

Comparison of Triage Systems

	TYPE I	TYPE II	TYPE III
ASSESSMENT	by receptionist, clerk, allied health personnel.	by RN or MD	by RN
	no data base, presenting complaint only.	limited data base; focus on chief complaint; including limited subjective and objective data	selected data base; including pertinent subjective and objective data, client education areas, primary health care needs.
PLAN	categories: —emergent —non-urgent	categories (based on care priorities) —emergent —urgent —delayed	categories (based on care priorities and reassessment needs): categories I-IV
	no determination of preliminary diagnostic procedures.	determination of selected diagnostic procedures.	determination of selected diagnostic procedures.
IMPLEMENTATION	sent to acute care or clinic waiting rooms.	directed to specific care area waiting room. MD may evaluate, treat and discharge in triage area.	directed to waiting area, reassessed every 15-60 minutes.
	no diagnostic procedures initiated.	diagnostic procedures initiated.	diagnostic procedures initiated.
	little or no documentation.	variable documentation.	systematic initial and ongoing documentation.
EVALUATION	client not evaluated again until treated.	no planned reevaluation. Client not evaluated again except as client requests reassessment or during diagnostic events.	scheduled reassessments of client according to standards.
	system evaluation difficult or impossible.	system evaluation variable.	built-in mechanisms for system evaluation.

Assessment

Client assessment is done by a receptionist, clerk or allied health personnel. No client data base is obtained; assessment consists solely of the chief complaint or "how sick" the client looks.

Plan and Implementation

Based on the triage agent's experience, the client is quickly judged to be "emergent" or "non-urgent." Acting as a traffic director the triage agent simply guides clients in the emergent category to one waiting or treatment area and those in the non-urgent category to another waiting area or clinic. No preliminary diagnostic procedures are determined or initiated.

Evaluation

The triage process ends when the client has been sent to the designated area. The individual is not evaluated again until actually treated. There is no opportunity for reassessment of the client or evaluation of changes in status. Documentation, at most, contains a statement of the client's chief complaint and destination. Consequently, ongoing evaluation of the triage process is difficult or impossible.

TYPE II—"SPOT CHECK"

The major intent of this type system is to establish priorities of care in order to ensure that immediate care is available for the most seriously ill or injured. Systems falling into this category include those termed "advanced triage."

Assessment

Client assessment is done by an RN or M.D. A selective data base is obtained including subjective and objective data about the client's chief complaint. Assessment focuses on the presenting complaint.

Plan

Based on the obtained data, clients are categorized according to levels of condition. The types of classification utilized vary; generally categories are based on both the urgency of the problem and a designated time frame. The following is a representative classification plan:

Emergent—life-threatening condition. The individual will die without immediate intervention.

Examples: ventricular cardiac arrhythmia, multiple trauma, massive head injuries, airway obstruction.

Urgent—conditions that require definitive management within 15 to 60 minutes.

Examples: open fractures, multiple lacerations, minor burns.

Delayed—conditions for which care can be delayed from four to six hours or longer.

Examples: sprains, fractures with minimal displacement.

Triage decisions are based on experience, and sometimes on written criteria or algorithms.

A determination of appropriate preliminary diagnostic procedures may be done by the triage person.

Implementation

The individual is categorized and directed to a specific care area. Triage notes consist of the assessment data and established category. Selected diagnostic procedures are initiated.

An M.D. carrying out triage may opt to evaluate, treat, and discharge a client in the triage area.

Evaluation

The triage process ends when the client is directed to the care area. The client is not evaluated again until treatment is initiated. Spot checks of client condition may occur during diagnosic events or at a client's request for reassessment.

The quality and type of documentation among Type II systems are variable; therefore, any triage system evaluation is equally variable.

TYPE III—"COMPREHENSIVE"

The major intent of this type of system is to utilize standards by which all clients will be assessed and reassessed by nursing personnel until the individual is medically evaluated. This section gives an overview of the Type III system. Chapter 4 discusses the system in detail. Part 2 of the text describes the implementation process for the Type III system.

Assessment

Client assessment is done by an RN. A client data base is obtained from subjective and objective data, which includes selective analysis of physical status, past history, history of present illness, review of systems, symptom analysis, social history, family history, health behaviors, and health hazards. This assessment, while comprehensive, must be condensed into a two- to five-minute period. It then provides a profile for the determination of immediate physiological needs, client or parent education needs, and selected primary health care needs.

Plan

Clients are categorized according to priorities based on the urgency of the condition and the need for reassessment. The following is the classification plan:

Category I—condition requires life-saving medical care.

Examples: seizures, multiple trauma

Category II—the condition is stable but care is needed as soon as space is available. The client will be reevaluated every 15 minutes until seen by an M.D. or recategorized.

Examples: probable extremity fracture, minor burn, history of sickle cell with client now experiencing pain.

Category III—the condition is stable and the individual is in no distress. The client will be reevaluated every 30 minutes until seen by an M.D. or recategorized.

Examples: non-bleeding laceration, drug ingestion more than three hours ago but client now showing no signs of distress.

Category IV—the condition is stable and the individual is in no distress. The client will be seen as space and medical personnel become available. The client will be reevaluated every 60 minutes until seen by an M.D. or recategorized.

Examples: rashes, constipation, "nerves."

Triage decisions are based upon experience and protocols. All triage nurses attend an educational program so that the protocols are similarly interpreted.

A determination of appropriate preliminary diagnostic procedures is done by the triage person using the protocol guidelines.

Implementation

The individual is categorized, assigned to a treatment area, and directed to a waiting area unless treated immediately. The individ-

CHARACTERISTIC	TYPE I	TYPE II	TYPE III
1. expedites client care through immediate assessment by the triage person.	Minimal		
2. provides the opportunity to develop a selected client data base.	Chief complaint only	Chief complaint, variable other data	Chief complaint, other data per protocol
3. ensures the establishment of client care priorities according to the acuteness of the conditions.			
4. decreases client delays by initiating diagnostic procedures.		Variable	Per protocol
5. provides continuous reassessment of individuals waiting for treatment.			
6. provides the opportunity to identify selected client or family health learning needs.			
7. functions as a screening area for individuals needing information.			
8. functions as a referral site for selected clients not requiring emergency care.			
9. relieves congestion in critical treatment areas and improves traffic flow through utilization of a variety of health care resources.	Minimal		
10. assists in effective utilization of space and personnel through the assignment of clients to designated treatment areas.		Variable	
11. promotes rapport through immediate demonstration of concern for emergency department client problems.			
12. has built-in mechanisms for continued system audit.		Variable	
13. decreases anxiety levels of client and family by providing immediate ongoing assessment while the client is waiting for medical care.			Probable
14. improves public relations by providing initial and continued client care "in the lobby."			Probable

Figure 3-1   Comparison of triage systems.

ual is reassessed by a triage nurse according to the specified standards.

Triage notes consist of the initial data base and reassessment data. Selected diagnostic procedures are initiated.

Evaluation

Every client is reassessed at least every 60 minutes and as frequently as every 15 minutes depending on his or her condition. Recategorization may occur at any time as changes in the client condition necessitate.

Ongoing evaluation of the triage process is facilitated by the consistent and systematic documentation procedure.

SUMMARY

To review the characteristics of a triage system as seen in Figure 3-1, only a Type III system fulfills all expectations of an effective and efficient system. A Type I system carries out triage only on a gross level and is minimally effective in expediting client care and relieving congestion. While a Type II system satisfies most of the functions, it has constraints in the areas of assessment, reassessment, and evaluation. The limited data base in a Type II system provides no opportunity for identification of client health and learning needs. Both areas are important for future health maintenance and prevention of emergency department visits. With client condition subject to rapid change, a Type II system provides no scheduled reassessment. At best, reevaluations may occur on a "spot check" basis. While evaluation of the triage process is feasible in a Type II system, it is dependent upon a standardized data collection and documentation system, which is highly variable in quality. One additional constraint in a Type II system occurs when treatment takes place in the triage area. Treatment impedes the triage process and makes it less efficient.

REFERENCES

Barber, Janet M., and Susan A. Budassi. Mosby's manual of emergency care practices and procedures, St. Louis, 1979: The C.V. Mosby Company, pp. 1-12.

Cosgriff, James, H., Jr., and Diann Laden Anderson. The practice of emergency nursing, New York, 1975: J.B. Lippincott Company, pp. 61-70.

Estrada, Elizabeth G: Advanced triage by an R.N., J.E.N., 5(6): pp. 15-18, November/December 1979.

McLeod, Kathryn: Part 1, Learning to take the trauma of triage, R.N. 38. pp. 22-27, July 1975.

Nelson, Doris M.: Triage and assessment, in Carmen G Warner, editor: Emergency care, assessment and intervention, ed. 5, St. Louis, 1978: The C.V. Mosby Company, pp. 45-57.

Nelson, Doris M.: Triage in the emergency suite, Hosp. Top., 51(9): pp. 39-41, September 1973.

Nyberg, Jan: Perception of patient problems in the emergency department, J.E.N., 84(1): pp. 15-19, January/February 1978.

Pool, Mickey: Triage nursing as problem solving, J.E.N., 2(6): pp. 25-27, November/December 1976.

Russo, Raymond M.: Ambulatory care triage, Am. Fam. Physician, 9(2): pp. 125-130, February 1974.

Slay, Larry E., and Wayne G. Riskin. Algorithm-directed triage in an emergency department, J.A.C.E.P., 5(11): pp. 869-876, November 1976.

Waeckerle, Joseph F., Michael Gaughan, Robert Billings, and W. Kendall McNabney. The emergency nurse as a primary health care provider, J.E.N., 3(4): pp. 21-25, July/August 1977.

Weinerman, E. Richard, and Herbert R. Edwards, 'Triage' system shows promise in management of emergency department load, Hospitals, 38(22): pp. 55-62, November 16, 1964.

Willis, Dorothy T.. A study of nursing triage, J.E.N., 5(6): pp. 8-11, November/December 1979.

Blueprint of a Comprehensive Triage System

Chapter 4

THE TYPE III SYSTEM

The proposed system provides quality health care "in the lobby" as well as defines the idea that the individual will be seen by the right person, in the right place, at the right time, for the right thing. The system ensures the separation and referral of persons based upon the type and severity of their condition.

THE TRIAGE SYSTEM BLUEPRINT

The Type III triage system has 11 major components. Following a brief listing of the steps each component will be described in detail. The steps of the triage process are:

1. Clients entering the emergency department are first assessed by the triage nurse. Those *critically* injured and ill clients are referred for immediate care.

29

2. During the assessment, each client is briefly subjectively and objectively evaluated. The client chart is initiated.

3. When necessary, appropriate splinting, bandaging, and other first aid techniques are applied. Children with high fevers may be treated with an antipyretic.

4. The appropriate x-ray and selective laboratory tests are initiated according to protocol.

5. The client is categorized according to the findings of the assessment. An arm band is applied. The client chart is marked with the appropriate categorization.

6. Depending upon the categorization, the client is either sent to the lobby to wait or to a room in the emergency department for immediate care.

7. Those clients returning to the lobby must go from the triage area to the traditional client registration area so that the business office data may be collected. Those clients requiring laboratory and x-ray studies must have all business office chart work completed prior to the clinical studies.

8. The clients then return to the lobby

9. The float nurse or the triage nurse provides continued assessment while the clients wait in the lobby. The clients receive either 15-minute, 30-minute, or 60-minute reassessment until they are seen by the physician. The type and frequency of assessment depends upon the client's categorization

10. The float nurse then determines who will go into an examination room next. It is the float nurse's responsibility to give report to the nurses "in the back." The float nurse is the "pulse" of the flow in the emergency department.

11. Clients may be recategorized at any time.

Figure 4-1 summarizes this triage process.

THE TRIAGE SYSTEM IN DETAIL

Triage Staffing

Depending upon the size of the emergency department and the client census, the staffing needs will obviously differ. Following are

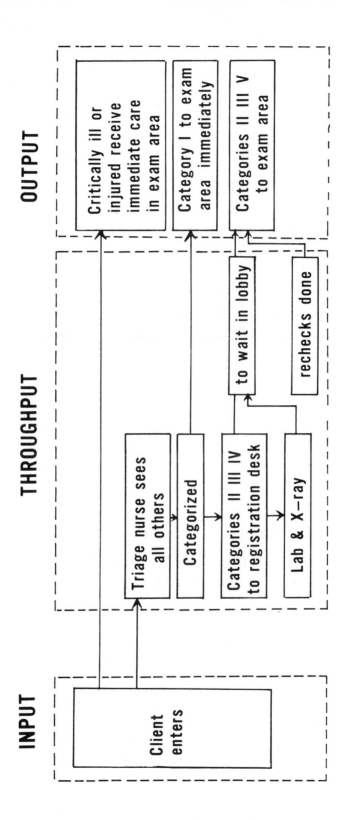

INPUT   THROUGHPUT   OUTPUT

Client enters

Triage nurse sees all others → Categorized

Categories II III IV to registration desk → Lab & X-ray

to wait in lobby

rechecks done

Critically ill or injured receive immediate care in exam area

Category I to exam area immediately

Categories II III V to exam area

Figure 4-1   The triage process.

31

the types of staff members found to be necessary in order to implement triage.

Triage Nurse

An RN who has completed the triage education program. This nurse is responsible for initially assessing all clients entering the emergency department. It is estimated that this nurse will spend between two to five minutes with each client.

Triage Nurse Helper

An ancillary worker assisting the triage nurse. This worker is responsible for implementing appropriate first aid techniques and measuring the vital signs. The ancillary worker actually works with the triage nurse to determine which of the incoming clients should be triaged next. Depending on the system, the ancillary worker may assist in collecting laboratory specimens and sending people to the x-ray department.

Float Nurse

An RN who has completed the triage education program. This nurse acts as the pulse of the triage system. The ultimate responsibilities include reassessing clients in the lobby, deciding who will be sent into examination room next, and giving a client assessment report to the nurses "in the back" when the client is placed in the examination room.

Triage Backup

An RN assigned as a backup to the triage system nurses. This person should respond to assist the system if it becomes bombarded with new clients. The backup nurse also rotates in the system for meals and time-out breaks.

As will be discussed in detail later, every RN staff member in the emergency department should go through the triage education program. Some staff members will enjoy triaging and others will not. The complexity of each system operations and the available staffing will determine whether or not a system is able to cater to staff member requests.

One of the major reasons staff members "do not like" to work triage is because it is an area of continued tension. Therefore, a two-hour rotational system for triage coverage may be useful. This not only provides a relief for the triage and float nurses, but also provides the opportunity for the triage nurses to follow clients once they have been triaged. Figure 4-2 illustrates two staff scheduling

R N Staffing for Triage Functioning

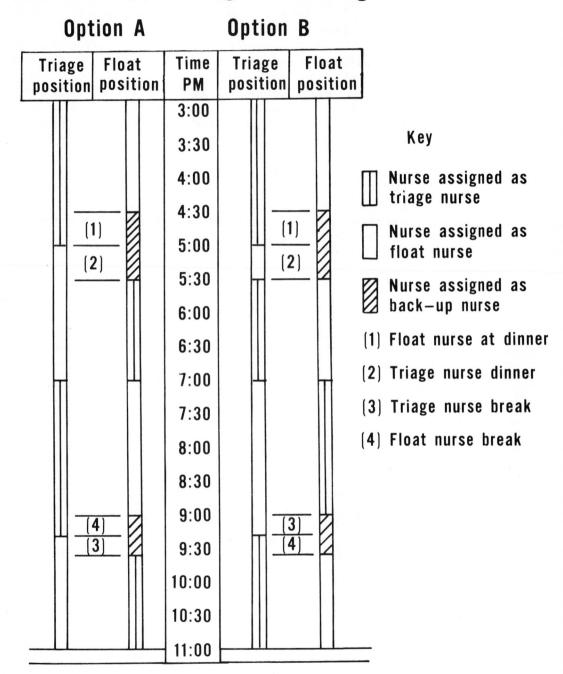

Figure 4-2 RN staffing for triage functioning.

examples. Note that three staff members are assigned to cover the two staffing positions (triage position, float position).

For less complex systems, it should be fairly easy to eliminate the ancillary worker. Whether or not the float nurse is eliminated is a more serious issue. While the triage nurse may be responsible for rechecking clients while they wait in the lobby, it is difficult for that nurse to also assess space availability "in the back." Therefore, if the float nurse is eliminated, someone "in the back" must continuously be in communication with the triage nurse to determine who should be seen next. Table 4-1 details three staffing variations, which are determined by estimated client flow through the department. The following table is based on the assumption that it will take approximately *five minutes* to initially assess and categorize each client. This time includes chart initiation, vital signs, and subjective and objective data collection. First aid treatment may extend beyond five minutes.

Table 4-1
Staffing Variations

HOSPITAL A		HOSPITAL B		HOSPITAL C	
Number of	150/shift	Number of	96/shift	Number of	60/shift
Clients	19/hour	Clients	12/hour	Clients	7.5/hour
1 client every 3 minutes		1 client every 5 minutes		1 client every 8 minutes	
2 triage nurses		1 triage nurse		1 triage nurse	
1 ancillary helper		1 ancillary helper		1 float nurse	
1 float nurse		1 float nurse		or	
				1 ancillary helper	

Discussion of how to determine staffing patterns will be detailed later. The important point to remember throughout this discussion is the simple fact that in order to implement an effective triage system the department will need more staff. It is impossible to expand quality services without increasing the number of persons to deliver those services.

Protocols for System Functioning

One of the major objectives of any triage system is to provide standardized quality care for all clients. To move toward a standardized system of client assessment, a complete set of assessment protocols based upon the client's chief complaint has been developed. These are discussed in detail in Part 3.

These protocols are most helpful in the education of the triage personnel. Staff members are required to assess each client in a similar format. Each protocol provides specific subjective and objective data and findings around which the triage nurse must make the client categorization decision. In the classroom setting, sample cases are studied as a means of utilizing the protocols. Through these case studies, the nurses should develop expertise in collecting the appropriate standardized data and making the correct categorization decision. In the actual triage setting, nurses should continue to collect the predetermined standardized data and make assessments to correctly categorize clients.

In the actual practice setting, the protocols are meant to provide support for the triage nurse's sorting decisions. While it is not likely that the nurse will "look up" the specific protocol for each client who is seen, the nurse must be extremely familiar with the protocols so that the appropriate categorizations are made. The protocols also provide specific information for appropriate x-ray and laboratory tests.

The protocols provide a standard upon which to evaluate the performance of the triage nurses and the categorization of the clients. The protocols are, therefore, quite assistive during chart audits, staff performance evaluation, and outcome audit.

The Client Encounter

Clients enter the emergency department on their own or by squad. The first health care professional to see the client is either the triage nurse, the float nurse, or the ancillary worker. The system is devised so that all three of the persons are stationed in the lobby area and near the front door.

A bird's-eye view assessment will be made to initially determine the severity of the client's solution. With the exception of a very few clients requiring immediate care, all clients are initially seen by the triage nurse. If the triage nurse is busy with client "A" at the exact moment that client "B" arrives, the ancillary personnel may start to assess the situation and provide initial first aid. The ancillary worker should interrupt the triage nurse if necessary.

The triage nurse's job is as follows:

1. Collect a detailed symptom analysis of the client's complaint.

2. Perform brief objective data collection as indicated per protocol and according to the presented subjective data.

3. Measure vital signs (may be done by ancillary personnel).

4. Administer appropriate first aid measures such as splint-

        ing or applying a dressing to a laceration (may be done by ancillary worker).

5. Order x-rays or laboratory studies as indicated by the established protocols.

6. Administer medications such as antipyretics as indicated by the triage protocols.

7. Initiate the client chart by writing the name, age, weight, and vital signs. The nurse must also briefly document subjective and objective data including the client's complaint and the findings from the triage assessment. First aid care is documented as well as any laboratory or x-ray orders.

8. X-ray requests are written by the triage nurse. The laboratory requests may be written by the ancillary personnel or the personnel at the registration desk.

9. The triage nurse categorizes the client. The appropriate color arm band is placed on the client's wrist. This arm band also includes the client's name and emergency department chart number.

10. The client's chart is marked with the appropriate categorization number and color coding mark and is then given to either the registration desk or the float nurse.

11. At this point, the float nurse becomes responsible for the clients, directing them to the reception area for further registration, to the x-ray department if necessary, or to the lobby (the ancillary personnel may assist).

The entire triage process should take no longer than *five minutes.* The Type III triage system is completely developed around a five-minute flow-through system. This time frame is realistic providing that there is adequate education of the triage nurses, and adequate support by ancillary personnel.

The Categorization of Clients

All clients processed through the triage system will be categorized by the triage nurse. The purpose of the categorization is to set standards by which all clients will be initially assessed and, if necessary, reassessed by nursing personnel until the client is seen by the designated care provider. There are four client categories. The second through fourth categories include reassessment criteria. This means that the client, while waiting in the lobby, will be periodically reassessed by a nurse until the client is put into an examination room in the emergency department and assessed by the physician. The categories are as follows:

Category I

The client's condition requires life saving medical care. The client is very briefly evaluated by the triage nurse and immediately sent to the major area of the emergency department.

EXAMPLES: Seizures, major burn over 10 percent body surface area, fractured femur, obvious respiratory distress, multiple trauma, cardiac arrest.

CLIENT IDENTIFICATION: The client will undoubtedly be admitted. The arm band should therefore be the client's admission band.

Category II

The client's condition is evaluated as stable but the client should receive physician assessment as soon as space in the emergency department becomes available.

REASSESSMENT: To evaluate continued stability, the client will be reevaluated by the triage personnel every *15 minutes* until placed in an examination room. Once in the examination room, the rechecks should continue every 15 minutes until the client is evaluated by the designated health care provider. The provider will generally be the physician.

EXAMPLES: Child with croupy cough but not in respiratory distress, probable extremity fracture (circulation intact distally), possible appendix, minor burn, history of sickle cell with client now having pain.

CLIENT IDENTIFICATION: The client receives a red arm band. A red dot indicating Category II is placed at the top of the chart.

Category III

The client's condition is stable and no obvious distress is noted.

REASSESSMENT: The client will be reevaluated by the triage personnel every *30 minutes* until placed in an examination room. Once in the examination room, rechecks should continue every 30 minutes until the client is medically evaluated.

NOTE: Any client may be recategorized either upward or downward based upon the reassessment data.

EXAMPLES: Simple non-bleeding lacerations, possible sexual assault more than 12 hours ago but less than 72 hours, puncture wounds, drug ingestion over 3 hours ago with client now showing no discomfort or distress signs.

CLIENT IDENTIFICATION: The client receives a blue arm band. A blue dot indicating Category III is placed at the top of the chart.

Category IV

The client's condition is stable. No distress is noted. The client will be seen as space and medical personnel become available.

REASSESSMENT: The client must be reevaluated every 60 minutes until seen by the designated health care provider or until recategorized.

EXAMPLES: "nerves," impetigo, rashes, abrasions, constipation, inability to urinate in the past 12 hours.

CLIENT IDENTIFICATION: The client receives an orange arm band. An orange dot indicating Category IV is placed at the top of the chart.

Dots and Arm Bands

Reference has been made to a variety of colored dots and arm bands that are used during the triage process (see Figure 4-3). The three colors already discussed include:

Red arm band and dot for Category II clients

Blue arm band and dot for Category III clients

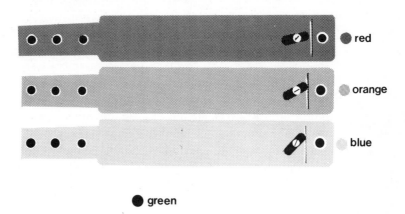

Figure 4-3   Identification materials for client categorization.

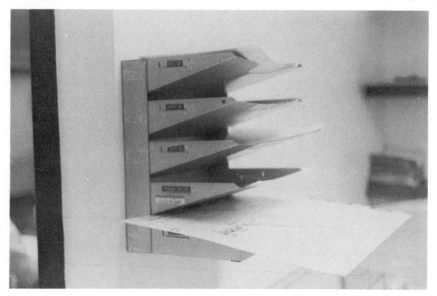

Figure 4-4   A rack designed to separate and prioritize charts.

Orange arm band and dot for Category IV clients

There is obviously nothing special about the colors stated here. What is important is that by using a variety of colors the categorization of the client is obvious for all personnel to see. The float nurse can view at a distance who the Category II clients are—thus, who needs frequent reassessment.

The colored dots on the charts likewise provide a visual sorting system as to the acuity of client problems. Again, the float nurse will find it quite helpful to quickly assess the acquired charts and to identify that, for example, two clients are Category II, four are Category III, and six are Category IV. The colored dots are simply visual cues for sorting and prioritizing the charts.

A chart rack such as seen in Figure 4-4 may be used by the float nurse to separate and prioritize the charts. This rack may be color coded into the three colors previously discussed.

Green Dot

The only dot that has not been discussed is the green dot (see Figure 4-3). This dot describes the need for further assessment or client education. In its purest sense, the green dot represents the nursing in triage. While the triage nurse is collecting the appropriate data to correctly categorize clients, data should also be collected about such things as the client's:

Regular primary care source

Completeness of immunizations

Knowledge about current health care problems

Knowledge about self-care as it relates to current problem

Primary health care needs

These are but a few of the categories of inquiry. The triage nurse must remain alert to the client's needs and should place a green dot on the chart with a brief note indicating the area of need. This dot then signals to the nurses "in the back" to follow up on that identified health care need.

During the brief encounter between the client and triage nurse, much data are collected. The triage nurse expands her sights beyond the categorization of the client to also identify other health care needs of the client. These may then be signaled by use of the green dot.

Completing the Chart

After the triage nurse has assessed and categorized the client, the chart and the client (or an appropriate family member) must go to the registration desk to complete the sign-in process. This is the traditional process where the client's address, insurance data, and signature are obtained. The chart is then given to the float nurse.

There are varying opinions as to whether it is necessary to obtain the client's or parent's signature for consent of treatment. These opinions range from "there is no need to obtain a signature at any time—because by the very fact that the client came to the emergency department, it is implied that treatment is requested" to "the signature must be obtained before any assessment is done." It is advised that this situation be discussed in your own institution and a decision made as to when during the triage process the signature is obtained. As indicated above, postponing the signature is advocated until the client officially signs in at the registration desk. This generally will be after the triage process but prior to x-ray, laboratory studies, or definitive treatment.

The Float Nurse and Client Reassessment

The float nurse has three primary responsibilities: first, client reassessment; second, room assignments in the examination area of the emergency department; and third, a report to the nurse "in the back" once the client is placed into a room.

Client Reassessment

The float nurse must reassess the clients at the designated 15-, 30-, and 60-minute intervals. The extent of the reassessment will depend upon the client's problems. Vital sign reassessments are determined on a case-by-case basis. The reassessment should be comprehensive enough to provide a continued update of the client's status.

In each case, the findings of the reassessment must be documented on the chart. Therefore, one would expect a Category II client to have a progress update written every 15 minutes.

The following are three reassessment examples:

1. Category II: Client with distal fracture of radius, splint in place, ice applied.
   Reassessment: Includes review of client's discomfort, objective assessment of radial pulse (compared to other wrist), color of hand, sensation to touch, ability to wiggle fingers.

2. Category III: Child with earache, fever on admission 102.6°, antipyretic given in triage.
   Reassessment: Includes review of client's discomfort and temperature reassessment after one-half hour.

3. Category II: Sixteen-year-old child in a bicycle accident, history of possible loss of consciousness. Client unable to recall events of accident. Vomited once prior to arrival in emergency department. Client appeared awake and alert during triage. Skull x-rays deferred until physician evaluation.
   Reassessment: Includes level of consciousness, vital signs, gross motor testing including client's ability to maintain position and move purposefully, history of additional vomiting.

Client Room Assignments

The float nurse should know which client in the lobby needs to be seen next. It is that nurse's responsibility to locate available examination room space and to move the clients back accordingly. If the condition of any client in the lobby deteriorates, the float nurse must communicate to the staff "in the back" the need for immediate space.

In a busy emergency department, Category IV clients may be

placed on "the back burner" and left sitting in the lobby for hours. The float nurse has the responsibility to slip these clients into the system at a steady pace so that they are not required to wait for hours on end.

Another option in many systems is for the Category IV clients to be sent to some type of ambulatory or minor medical clinic area. It is again up to the float nurse to make these referrals and to make sure that the client is directed to the appropriate area.

Report

When the client is placed in an examination room, the float nurse must give a report to the nurse receiving the client. This provides continuity of the care, which was started as the client entered the front doors of the emergency department. It is the firm belief of these authors that every emergency department must organize its nursing staff in a manner so that *each client has a designated nurse* who is responsible for planning and implementing the required care.

The Nurse in the Back

Once the nurse in the examination area receives the client from the float nurse, it becomes that nurse's responsibility to continue the client's care. That nurse must periodically reassess the client according to the predetermined criteria. These rechecks continue until the nurse determines a recategorization status or until the client is seen by the physician.

Triage System Space

It has been determined that the triage of clients occurs "in the lobby." The scope of this assessment will depend on the structural boundaries of each emergency department. In order to implement a comprehensive triage system, some structural changes may be necessary.

Prior to discussing structural plans, it is essential to consider what a *good* triage facility needs:

1. A place to interview the client. Only limited interviewing can be done at a desk in the emergency department waiting room or the hall. Some privacy is necessary.

2. Visual access to the emergency department entrance by the triage nurse so that each client entering the department can be seen.

3. A stretcher for clients requiring a place to lie down. This stretcher should provide some degree of privacy for the client. It is not to be used as a holding area but primarily as first aid space. The stretcher is also extremely useful for children requiring rectal temperatures and for clients with lower limb injuries.

4. A supply of splints, first aid materials, and selected medications. Included in this category should be ice bags, a small scrub sink, emesis basins, and bandaging supplies.

5. A vital sign area, including electronic equipment that facilitates rapid measurement of vital signs. Weight measurement should also be done.

6. Adequate space and privacy so that several staff members can work simultaneously if necessary.

7. Access of the triage center to the emergency department waiting room, the registration desk, and the internal emergency department.

Figures 4-5 through 4-8 depict the facility characteristics as stated above.

In order to implement a comprehensive triage system, some

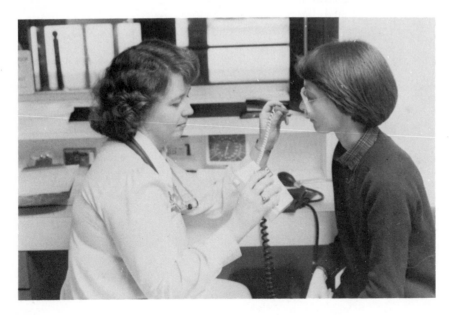

Figure 4-5a An example of a good interview and vital sign area.

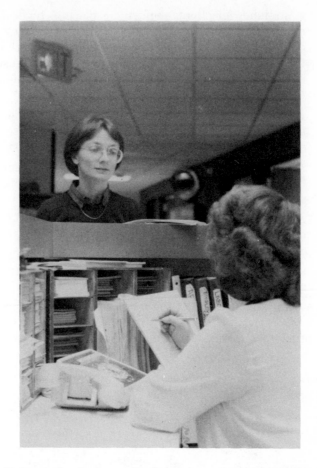

Figure 4-5b   An example of poor interview arrangements.

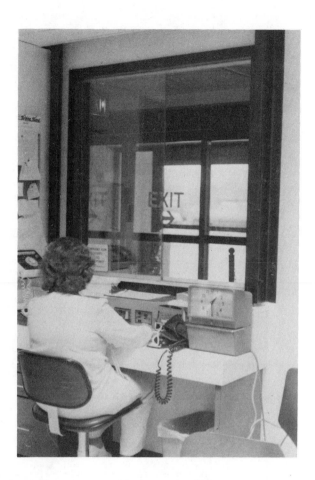

Figure 4-6 Visual access to the emergency department by the triage nurse.

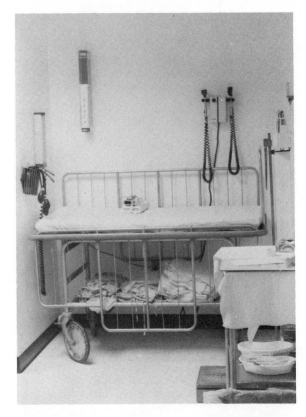

Figure 4-7　Privacy area within the triage center.

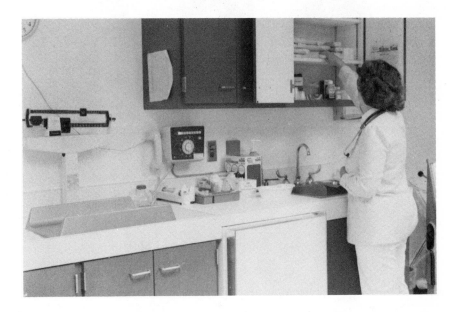

　Figure 4-8a　Supply area within the triage center.

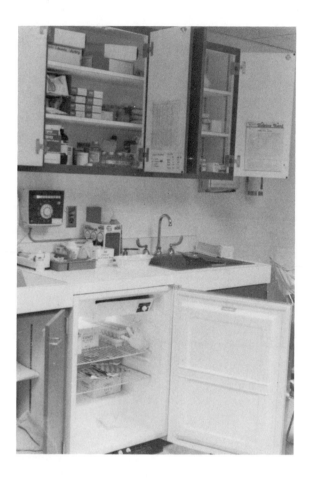

Figure 4-8b   Supply area within the triage center.

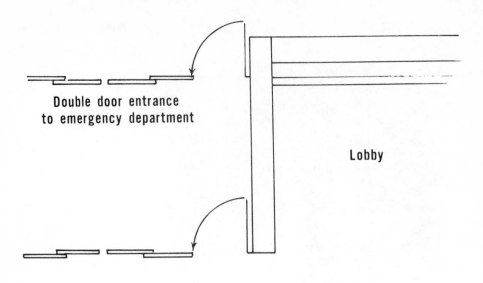

Double door entrance
to emergency department

Lobby

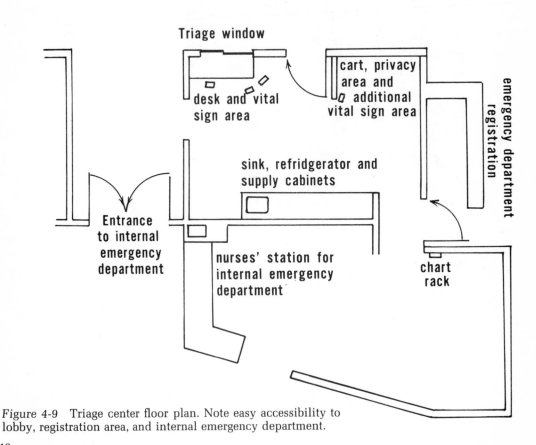

Triage window

desk and vital
sign area

cart, privacy
area and
additional
vital sign area

emergency department
registration

sink, refridgerator and
supply cabinets

Entrance
to internal
emergency
department

nurses' station for
internal emergency
department

chart
rack

Figure 4-9   Triage center floor plan. Note easy accessibility to
lobby, registration area, and internal emergency department.

type of structural remodeling will probably be necessary. The extent of that renovation will depend upon: (1) the volume of clients seen in the emergency department; (2) the anticipated staffing of the triage system; and (3) the scope of care offered during triage.

Figure 4-9 details the floor plan of a spacious triage center. This plan incorporates the seven necessary characteristics as stated previously. This model facility was constructed and is in operation at the Children's Hospital in Columbus, Ohio.

Evaluation of the Triage System

Chapter 5

Evaluation of the triage system is an ongoing appraisal of what the system does, how it does it, and how well it works. Evaluation is the process that ensures feedback into the system. Feedback provides information about the effectiveness and efficiency of the system. Such feedback is essential for the viability of the system and will provide the data necessary for system revisions and, thus, quality assurance.

System evaluation encompasses three components: structure, process, outcome. All three are essential for quality assurance. Each requires use of methods appropriate to it, with the understanding that each influences and may overlap the other two.

For the purposes of clarity and ease of discussion, each of these components will be discussed separately. Ultimately, however, none of the components should be considered exclusively from the others; it is the combination of all three that comprises full evaluation.

STRUCTURE EVALUATION

The structural components of space, equipment, and physical set-up were discussed in Chapter 4. While space allocation and architectural changes tend to be more permanent, there needs to be continued evaluation of the appropriateness of the equipment in use, the placement of such equipment, and the utilization of the available space. All triage personnel are appropriate agents for evaluation of these factors.

Another major structural component is that of staffing and staffing patterns. Staffing options have been presented in Chapter 4. The program planner may need to adapt these patterns to meet the special needs of each emergency department. It is critical that staffing remain stable and consistent. Without adequate and appropriate personnel to work the system, it will inevitably fail. There needs to be continuous evaluation from the triage agents as to how well the staffing patterns are working and where changes need to be made. Identification of peak and slow times will affect the staffing patterns.

The stress associated with performing triage is a structural component. Some of this stress can be alleviated or eliminated through use of the staffing patterns which build in limited periods of actual triage function alternated with the reassessment function of the float position. Other sources and areas of stress need to be identified and evaluated by the triage nurses. A decision maker under stress may well be a poor decision maker. This may ultimately affect the functioning and overall success of the entire triage system.

The client care protocols are a structural component that require ongoing evaluation. The triage personnel using the protocols should provide input to assess the following areas:

1.   Are the protocols sufficiently in-depth?
2.   Do more content areas need to be designed? What areas?
3.   How are the protocols being used?
4.   Was there adequate preparation for use of the protocols?
5.   What are the areas of difficulty?

Data from this evaluation will be used to make changes in the protocols and will also be fed back into the triage education program.

Methods for evaluation of structural components include formal or informal meetings and conferences with triage personnel on either an individual or group basis. Special times should be set aside to discuss the various evaluation areas. A retrospective technique can be utilized through discussion or questionnaires. A concurrent evaluation may occur through the use of a journal, checklist or other evaluation tool. A combination of methods will produce the most valid and reliable data.

PROCESS EVALUATION

Process evaluation deals with the activities of the triage system and essentially looks at everything that happens during the triage process. It evaluates the significant steps, the sequence of steps, and the degree to which these help achieve the goal of triage.

A major component to be evaluated is time. A time study should be undertaken to determine:

1. Time between emergency department arrival and triage assessment.
2. Time between triage assessment and room assignment.
3. Time between room assignment and physician evaluation.
4. Time discharged.

Variables that influence the amount of time spent in the emergency department also need to be considered. These may include such things as the amount of traffic through the department (peak/slow times), initiation of diagnostic tests performed in triage, the type and amount of diagnostic testing done, and the time spent waiting for physician consultants.

The number and nature of client-related incidents need to be continually monitored. Such incidents include client complaints about perceived delays in treatment or insufficient concern by staff, incident reports resulting from inappropriate delay in treatment, and the number of clients leaving against medical advice prior to initiation of physician care.

Traffic patterns and client flow through the emergency department are components of the process evaluation. Reports indicate that congestion and confusion are relieved in emergency departments with triage systems. The particular traffic patterns and flow for each facility should be assessed in the following areas:

1. Do triage personnel have easy access to waiting clients?
2. Is client routing satisfactory?
3. Is traffic flowing in multiple directions in any one area?
4. Is there immediate access to treatment areas for Category I clients?
5. What are the times when—or areas where—clients get backed up?
6. Are chairs in the waiting area conveniently arranged for clients and triage nurses?

7.   Are waiting areas crowded?

Multiple sources can be used to obtain data for the process evaluation. The client record should be a source of data for the time study. The records utilized in the Type III system should have provisions for the notations of time. Triage and other emergency department personnel can provide input in the other areas of evaluation. Clients may provide useful insights regarding traffic patterns and flow.

Appropriate methods for evaluation include interviews, questionnaires, participant observation, and non-participant observation.

OUTCOME EVALUATION

The effectiveness of the triage system is measured through its end results. In the evaluation of the triage system, four areas of outcome must be considered:

1.   The client assessment.
2.   The distribution of triage decisions.
3.   The accuracy of triage decisions and referrals.
4.   Client and community satisfaction.

A retrospective chart audit is a recommended methodology for evaluation of the first three areas listed above. Retrospective evaluation permits a reflective examination of completed cycles of the triage process and identification of achievements, trends, and problems by using randomized samples of client care records. The client records utilized in the Type III system facilitate the evaluation of assessment, reassessment, and disposition. The evaluation committee should be comprised of both physicians and nurses.

Client Assessments

Client assessment is the critical first step in the triage process. The rest of the process flows from these assessments. Continual evaluation of the assessment process is necessary in order to maintain high level assessment and, hence, high level triage.

The client record should be evaluated for the following:

1.   The type and quality of information recorded.
    a.   Consistency with protocols.
    b.   Missing data.
    c.   Amount of data—too much, too little.
    d.   Correctness of diagnostic tests initiated.

2. Consistency of documentation—with both initial and reassessment data.
3. The amount of time spent in assessment.

Findings from this evaluation should be fed back into the triage system and education program so that appropriate changes can be made.

Distribution of Triage Decisions

Evaluation in this area is directed toward the number of clients assigned to each category, the trends in category assignment, and the number of clients referred to other resources. This evaluation will provide information about utilization of alternate resources and reduction of daily client load.

The use of the emergency department for non-emergent problems has previously been discussed. The function of separating out those individuals not requiring emergency care subsequently reduces the client load. This, in turn, facilitates the care process.

Data from this evaluation can also be considered in assessing how the protocols are being used in making category decisions and assignments.

Accuracy of Triage Decisions and Referrals

Triage decisions are considered accurate or correct if there is evaluator agreement on the appropriateness of the categorization decision. The established protocols serve as guidelines for the evaluators. Mistriage occurs when evaluators agree that the case was less serious than triaged (up-triage) or more serious than triaged (down-triage).

Triage referrals can be evaluated in the same manner, through evaluator agreement in the appropriateness of the referral.

Variables affecting the interpretation of the triage and referral decisions need to be identified. An example is deliberate mis-referral in instances when such a decision expedites care. These variables will be specific to each institution.

Findings from this area of evaluation will contribute information pertinent to evaluation of the protocols and to the triage education program.

Client and Community Satisfaction

To be successful, a system needs to "satisfy its customer." In this case, the customer is the individual client and the community as a whole. Client assessment of the system alerts the triage personnel to the public's perception of them. Additionally, data can indicate if, or how well, the system is fulfilling its purpose. The value of client feedback is the identification of client satisfaction or the areas for improvement.

Client evaluation of the system may be carried out in a number of ways: directly, through questionnaires and interviews, or indirectly, through suggestion boxes, incident reports, and the news media.

SUMMARY

Evaluation is a time- and energy-consuming undertaking. Standards for evaluation must be developed that are specific to each institution and client population. Methodologies for evaluation have been suggested. These need to be adapted for the particular needs and situation of each emergency department. The process is continuous and requires commitment from everyone participating in it. As involved as evaluation may be, it is essential for the successful, effective, and efficient functioning of the triage system.

REFERENCES

Albin, Susan L., S. Wassertheil-Smoller, S. Jacobson, and B. Bell. Evaluation of emergency room triage performed by nurses, Am. J. Public Health, 65(10): pp. 1063–1068, October 1975.

Cayten, C. Gene and William Evans. Severity indices and their implications for emergency medical services research and evaluation, J. Trauma, 19(2): pp. 98–102, February 1979.

DeAngelis, Catherine and Margaret McHugh. The effectiveness of various health personnel as triage agents, J. Community Health, 2(4): 268–277, Summer 1977.

Froebe, Doris J., and R. Joyce Bain. Quality assurance programs and controls in nursing, St. Louis, 1976: The C.V. Mosby Company.

Gibson, Geoffrey. The emergency department as a screening point for hospital specialty services: inclusionary versus exclusionary strategies, Soc. Sci. Med., 13A(4): pp. 495–498, 1979.

Mills, J., Anna L. Webster, Constance B. Wofsy, P. Harding, and Donna D'Acuti. Effectiveness of nurse triage in the emergency department of an urban county hospital, J.A.C.E.P., 5(11): pp. 877–882, November 1976.

Phaneuf, Maria C. The nursing audit, ed. 2, New York, 1976: Appleton-Century-Crofts.

Russo, Raymond M. Ambulatory care triage, Am. Fam. Physician, 9(2): pp. 125–130, February 1974.

Slater, Reda R. Triage nurse in the emergency department, Am. J. Nurs., 70(1): pp. 127–129, January 1970.

Weinerman, E. Richard, and Herbert R. Edwards. 'Triage' system shows promise in management of emergency department load, Hospitals, 38(22): pp. 55–62, November 16, 1964.

Willis, Dorothy T. A study of nursing triage, J.E.N., 5(6): pp. 8–11, Novem-December 1979.

Legal Implications
In Triage

Chapter 6

LEGAL LIABILITY

Triage in the emergency department is now expected to be a nursing function. Placing the function of triage in the domain of nursing increases the professional responsibility of emergency nurses. With this increased authority and responsibility comes increased accountability and liability. A fundamental precept of the legal system is that each individual is personally responsible for his or her own acts. Triage nurses are, therefore, legally responsible for their own actions. In order to minimize legal liability for the triage nurse, systems should be developed that incorporate the following:

1. Availability of physician consultation with the triage nurses.

2. Structured educational programs for triage personnel.

3. Criteria guidelines for prioritization of client problems.

ASSESSMENT

Assessment as a professional act implies the exercise of judgment. This means the observation and evaluation of significant changes in a client's physical condition or the determination of the relative significance of a client's verbal complaints. Nursing judgment is inextricably involved in the process of triage. In assessing the client's need for emergency care, including the initial and follow-up assessments, the triage agent should act in accordance with accepted nursing standards. Triage in the emergency department is a specialized function that requires specialized guidelines and skills. A triage education program with ongoing evaluation is, therefore, essential to maintain the level of triage functioning that is compatible with the predetermined nursing standards.

Adherence to accepted standards should result in what is legally established as a fundamental rule of liability in client care: reasonable care under the circumstances. Any one of several triage decisions could be legally justified if it demonstrates that the nurse exercised reasonable care under the circumstances. The established protocols for gathering data and for categorization will assist the triage nurse to make triage decisions based upon appropriate information, and in accordance with accepted standards.

FACILITATION OF TREATMENT

In performing triage, the nurse will determine the order in which clients are treated. Each client has the right to physician care even though the nurse may believe no emergency exists. In situations where there is doubt whether an emergency exists, the doubt will be construed in favor of the client. The client's physical presence in the emergency department presumes that an emergency condition exists. Turning a client away may violate the law, depending on the state. Some states have laws and regulations that underscore the rights of emergency department clients ultimately to be evaluated and treated by the emergency physician (George, 1979)

In instances when a client is waiting for a private physician, appropriate triage and treatment measures need to be carried out while efforts are made to contact the physician. In no circumstances should necessary treatment be delayed because the private physician cannot be located. Nor should the triage agent be swayed by the client's statement of "I'm okay. I'll just wait." Such a comment is not accepted as a definitive state of the client's condition (George, 1980).

A client who refuses triage intervention, treatment, or diagnostic measures should be asked to sign a form of refusal, which should be witnessed. If the client refuses to sign, that refusal should be recorded on the form and witnessed. A client who chooses to leave the emergency department prior to treatment should be asked to sign a release form indicating the individual's decision to leave against medical advice (AMA).

TELEPHONE TRIAGE

Clients may call the emergency department with a variety of questions requesting advice and telephone treatment. While this is convenient for the client, it is legally hazardous for the triage agent. The general rule for telephone triage is to instruct the client to come to the emergency department for evaluation. No determination of the client's condition can be safely made without seeing the individual, regardless of how well that person describes the symptoms and problem. If a client dies or is injured as a result of telephone advice, the hospital and the person giving that advice may be held liable. The best way of handling telephone triage is to tell the client, "We cannot diagnose your problem over the phone. If you come in, we will be happy to treat you" (George, 1980).

An additional risk in giving telephone advice is that nurses may be charged with going beyond the scope of their practice. Such advice may be interpreted as practicing medicine and would thereby be in violation of the state medical or nurse practice act. This violation would be grounds for a negligence suit and would open the possibility of license suspension or revocation (George, 1980).

COMMUNICATION

Professional assessment implies that something meaningful will be done once the assessment is made. Communication, which includes documentation, is an integral part of assessment, at least from the legal standpoint (Regan, 1980). Effective communication must take place between the triage nurse and the staff in the back, and with other departments in the hospital.

Client records are an essential component of the communication aspect and also provide documentation. Accurate documentation is indispensable for legal purposes and in compensation cases. The triage notes should be a permanent part of the client's emergency department record, and should contain the following:

1. Client identification
2. Information concerning the arrival and means of arrival
3. Time of admission and discharge
4. Pertinent subjective and objective data about the injury or illness
5. Significant clinical, lab, or x-ray data
6. Categorization
7. First aid treatment
8. Reassessment data according to the predetermined criterial and time intervals
9. Final disposition
10. Signature of triage nurse

SUMMARY

Increased professional responsibility carries with it increased accountability and liability. The triage nurse faces legal accountability in several areas: assessment, facilitation of treatment, telephone triage, and communication. Basic legal precepts offer guidelines for action in those situations:

1. Personal responsibility for one's own acts
2. Reasonable care under the circumstances
3. Care in accordance with accepted standards

In designing and implementing a triage system, the program coordinator needs to pay special attention to certain J.C.A.H. (Joint Commission on Accreditation of Hospitals) Standards for Emergency Services. Standard II addresses staffing and specifies that there should be an adequate number of nurses for the amount and type of care to be provided. It further specifies the need for special training and for possession of professional skills for adequate performance of the duties. This can be fulfilled through the triage education program delineated in this book along with the guidelines for staffing. Standard IV addresses the need for written policies and procedures, which can be fulfilled, in part, by the triage protocols established in this text. Standard V provides for a client record, which has been addressed both in this chapter and in Chapter 4. Adherence to these standards can assist in maintaining high quality services and decrease the liability of the triage function.

REFERENCES

Creighton, Helen. Law for the nurse supervisor, emergency services management, Supervisor Nurse, 9: pp. 60-68, August 1978.

Creighton, Helen. Your legal risks in emergency care, Nursing '78, 8: pp. 52-55, February 1978.

George, James E., editor. Emergency nurse triage—beware, Emergency Nurse Legal Bulletin, 2(1): pp. 6-10, Winter 1976.

George, James E. Law and emergency care, St. Louis, 1980: The C.V. Mosby Company, pp. 66-78, 122, 133.

George, James E., editor. Triage—perils and pitfalls, Emergency Nurse Legal Bulletin, 5(2): pp. 2-8, Spring 1979.

Joint Commission on Accreditation of Hospitals: Accreditation manual for hospitals, 1980 ed., Chicago, 1980, pp. 23-34.

Regan, William, editor. Emergency care: reasonable limit on liability, Regan Report on Nursing Law, 17(4), September 1976.

Regan, William, editor. Nursing assessment: legal impact, Regan Report on Nursing Law, 21(2), July 1980.

Regan, William, editor. Nursing judgment: professional hallmark, Regan Report on Nursing Law, 18(9), February 1978.

The Implementation Process for a Comprehensive Triage System

Part 2

Who's Who in System Assessment

Chapter 7

An important first step in implementing a comprehensive triage system is to identify the types of individuals in the system who are affected by the triage program. By reconstructing the systems model diagram from Chapter 1 (see Table 7-1), *several* personnel groups should be anticipated. It is important for the program planner to consider the players and the role played by each.

The identified personnel groups as discussed in this chapter are only an example of all possible persons. Each program planner must search through the designated hospital system to identify the significant persons. The hospital's administrative structure and the type of emergency department physician coverage are variables in determining the "who's who."

Following is a detailed description of persons who are commonly identified as participants in hospital triage systems. For each group, the following areas will be discussed: involvement criteria in the triage system, anticipated resistance factors, anticipated educational needs, and the anticipated extent of the group's involvement in the triage plans and implementation.

NURSING STAFF

Registered Nurses

How Involved

This group is the primary target for system implementation. These are the individuals who perform triage. The program planner must establish the support of this group early and involve them in most of the steps in triage planning.

Anticipated Resistance Factors

Three primary resistance factors have been identified:

1. Value incongruency: Most nurses practicing in emergency departments choose that area of practice because of the challenges and excitement of trauma and lifesaving techniques. Triage, to some of these nurses, may be viewed as "boring," "hand holding," or just plain "stupid." Other nurses view triage as a real opportunity to get to know the clients, to implement primary nursing management, and to provide better initial client assessment and care. The preference of the emergency department nursing staff becomes apparent fairly quickly.

    These authors are not convinced that every nurse must be totally involved in the triage system. If there are selected nurses who enjoy triage, then it is advantageous to heavily involve those persons. If the emergency department staff is very small, then perhaps it is necessary for all nurses to become "triage nurses." If the emergency department nursing staff is large and all nurses are not involved in triage, there is an increased potential for program resistance or sabotage. Most resistance comes from ignorance of the potential scope of or a difference in values in the triage process. It is, therefore, vitally important to provide triage system education for all registered nurses in the department.

2. Non-involvement in planning: A second type of nurse resistance comes from not involving the staff in program planning early enough. A comprehensive triage system requires the total support of each implementer. It is vitally important that the registered nurse staff is involved early in concept and detail development. This will be further discussed in Chapter 8.

3. Past experience: The third type of anticipated resistance may be from nurses who have worked in other hospital systems where a poor triage system was implemented. There are many poorly implemented triage systems in operation today that are very boring for the nurse. Many of these do not require intellectual processing of client problems, and may include little or no nursing care. Again, the key to avoiding this resistance factor is early involvement of staff nurses and continual education for unfreezing.

Anticipated Educational Needs

There are three areas of required education:

1. The scope of the triage process: This should include the discussion of the expanded role of nursing in the early assessment and care of clients. In a well-planned and implemented triage system, the scope of responsibilities of nursing is greatly expanded.

2. The anticipated triage plan: All nurses need to be exposed to this very early. The program planner must be very assertive when proposing the system and the scope of the triage process. It is following this introduction that the program planner works with staff members to individualize the plan for that particular institution. This is the beginning of unfreezing and is discussed in more detail in Chapters 8 and 9.

3. The actual triage process: This is the most specific type of education required for all registered nurses in the emergency department. The nurses *must* receive standardized education in a formally planned program. The nurses must be taught to collect uniform subjective and objective client data, which will consistently result in similar assessments. Chapter 12 details the proposed educational program. All education is centered around the standardized use of the client protocols in Part 3 of this text.

    Perhaps one of the most important considerations for the program planner is to decide who should be educated. Should it be all registered nurses? Only those nurses who will be actually involved in triaging? Should trauma nurses and those who have been in the department less than two years be excluded? The answer to these and similar questions must be settled on an individual hospital basis. The education of all registered nurses in the department is advocated so that each will better understand the scope and responsibilities of the triage nurse.

Extent of Planning and Implementation Involvement

Registered nurses are the target group for planning and implementing. They should, therefore, be involved very early when triage is still in its conceptual form. Involvement continues through the specific system planning, implementation, and evaluation. Once the system is functional, the involved staff should be the primary group to implement the system's ongoing evaluation and appropriate revisions.

Licensed Practical Nurses or Licensed Vocational Nurses

How Involved

While the use of LPNs or LVNs in the actual triage process is not advocated, they are members of the emergency department team and may be involved in the reassessment process. As clients are assigned to examining rooms, the LPNs and LVNs may assume the function of client re-evaluation until the client is seen by the physician.

Anticipated Resistance Factors

Major resistance is most likely to surface from the issue that LPNs and LVNs do not act as triage nurses. While these authors sympathize with this position, we maintain that because of the legal restrictions and the practice liability of triaging, the triage process is outside of the scope of practice of the LVN or LPN. Practice codes for LPNs and LVNs state they practice nursing "at the direction of" a variety of health care providers including the registered nurse. It is, therefore, inappropriate to place an LPN or an LVN in a position of independent and critical decision making about client care.

Anticipated Educational Needs

These nurses require information about the triage system as a process, and their involvement in it. Careful and complete explanation must be made as to who's who in the triage process and the functions of each team member. LPNs and LVNs are team members in that they care for those clients who have been triaged. They must thoroughly understand the categorization criteria and the implications for client re-evaluation. They are also responsible in conjunction with the RNs for following through on client education and follow-up needs.

Extent of Planning and Implementation Involvement

LPNs and LVNs are not directly involved in the planning of the triage system. They should be continually informed of the triage plans and their role in the implementation of the program. It is imperative that these staff members be kept informed as the program plans develop.

PHYSICIAN STAFF

Permanent Emergency Department Physician Staff

How Involved

The triage program "belongs" to this group of staff members equally with the registered nurse group. The physician group must endorse the triage concept prior to any extensive program planning. The program planner should work closely with this group as the client protocols are being developed.

The physicians must thoroughly understand and agree with the categorization criteria. It is important to present completed program plans to this group for final approval. If the program planner has worked closely with the physician group as the program was being developed, the final approval should be easily obtained.

If there are multiple physicians involved, it is advantageous to designate a single physician as the primary consultant to the triage project. This physician consultant should hold enough authority so that as items are approved, other physician endorsement will follow.

Anticipated Resistance Factors

Resistance may stem from the concern that nurses are assuming more responsibility than they should; that nurses are ordering x-ray and laboratory studies; and that triage slows client care. Obviously, if clients would enter an emergency department at a pace that would allow immediate care by a physician, then triage would not be necessary. However, the increasing numbers of clients as documented in Chapter 2 have caused backlogs of clients waiting to be seen. Certainly, a comprehensive service that provides initial diagnostic data for the physician to consider is helpful in providing quality and efficient client care.

Anticipated Educational Needs

There are two specific educational needs for physicians:

1. Clarification of the purpose and function of the triage process so that role misunderstanding does not occur. The program planner must facilitate understanding so that the physicians do not regard the triage nurse function as an attempt to usurp the physician role. Nurses, as members of the health care team, are trying to ensure quality and expedite care so that the right client is seen in the right place, by the right person, at the right time for the right thing. Triage is a method by which to improve client care and satisfaction. Both elements are important to the emergency care team.

2. Explanation of the protocols: The physician staff must understand the approved protocols, the basic categorization criteria, and the process for rechecks. This education can be accomplished during a staff conference prior to the initiation of the triage program.

Extent of Planning and Implementation Involvement

As discussed earlier, one physician should be designated to work closely with the program planner. Once the program plans and protocols are developed, the materials should be discussed with the physician consultant for review and approval. Following this approval, the plans and protocols should be submitted to the larger physician group for endorsement.

Once the program is operational, it is very important to continue program evaluation with the involved physicians. The efficient and effective functioning of the triage process depends upon total team cooperation and review.

House Staff

How Involved

Due to the limitations imposed by the rotation of these physicians through the emergency department, their involvement in the triage process and planning is peripheral. Their involvement extends only to the reception of the assessed and categorized clients.

Anticipated Resistance Factors

As the program is implemented, the house staff may have the same resistance as the staff physicians. Once the program is operational, however, resistance should decrease and will vary from individual to individual.

Anticipated Educational Needs

The house staff require basic education about the program, including the process of initial assessment and the purpose of categorization and reassessment. This should be a factual presentation as part of their overall unit orientation.

Extent of Planning and Implementation Involvement

House staff members should not play a role in planning the triage system.

Community Physicians

How Involved

Community physicians are involved to differing degrees depending on their practice privileges and responsibilities in the emergency department. All physicians who send their clients to the emergency department or who utilize the emergency department should be informed of the process.

Anticipated Resistance Factors

Resistance will most likely stem from lack of information. Once the community physicians are informed of the process, they are generally supportive and appreciate the prompt client assessment and reassessment while they reach the hospital.

Anticipated Educational Needs

These physicians need to be educated about the need and purpose of the triage system. They need to understand how clients will be assessed and categorized.

Extent of Planning and Implementation Involvement

Community physicians should not be involved in the planning of the triage system. If the facility has special privileges for private physicians, then the details of those privileges and the procedure for the triage of their clients must be negotiated.

OTHER EMERGENCY DEPARTMENT STAFF

Ancillary Staff

This group consists of aides, orderlies, paramedics, and nursing students.

How Involved

This group of personnel is directly involved in the triage process by assisting with first aid, vital signs, and weight assessments with the triage nurse, or with reassessments with the float nurse.

Anticipated Resistance Factors

There are two anticipated resistance factors:

1. Monotony and boredom with the required job: This is a valid point that must be anticipated and dealt with. The best negotiation strategy is to develop an ancillary rotation schedule so that staff members will not be required to work in the positions for more than two hours at a single interval. Nursing students working in the emergency department as nursing assistants consider working in the ancillary triage position challenging. They are able to work side-by-side with the triage and float nurses and seem to reap many benefits and deliver a valuable service.

2. Ancillary staff role change: This second resistance point may be seen if the personnel had assumed the role as an informal triage agent prior to this formalized program. If this is the case, the ancillary staff may perceive that their work is no longer valued or needed. This is reinforced by their new assignment of vital signs assessor. It is vitally important for the program planner to evaluate this possible resistance and to discuss its significance with the involved staff members. Sometimes openness and honesty help in reducing the resistance.

Anticipated Educational Needs

Like the LPNs and LVNs, ancillary workers require information about the triage system as a process and their involvement in it. They need specific information about appropriate first aid to be applied in triage, techniques for obtaining vital signs, and how to work cooperatively with the triage and float nurses.

Ancillary workers are a vital part of the successful triage implementation. The program should begin early in informing this group of the proposed triage plans and their role in the triage process.

Extent of Planning and Implementation Involvement

Ancillary staffers are not directly involved in the triage program plans. They must be kept informed of the plans and their anticipated role in the program implementation. Once the program is operational, ancillary workers should be involved in the ongoing evaluation process.

Ward Clerks or Business Office Clerks

Ward clerks or business office clerks in most hospitals have been the informal triage agents for many years. In the comprehensive triage system, they are being relieved of this stressful position and may return to perform the duties for which they were hired.

How Involved

In the proposed system, the ward clerks or business office clerks see the client or the client's family after the client has been assessed by the triage nurse. The clerks no longer initiate the client's record. This necessitates education about their altered role and function.

Anticipated Resistance Factors

Resistance may occur if the clerks are not adequately informed about the new system. There are distinct changes in their roles and they must be informed as to why they are being "relieved" of their triage function and why the chart is being initiated by the triage nurse.

Anticipated Educational Needs

Several meetings should be scheduled with the clerks. They need information about the proposed system and their specific roles in that program's implementation.

If the triage program is not to be operational 24 hours a day, the clerks must be informed as to their specific roles during the triage system's shutdown period.

Extent of Planning and Implementation Involvement

The program planner should work closely with the clerks to determine stressful areas as the system is actually implemented.

HOSPITAL ADMINISTRATION

It is difficult to anticipate all the individuals who must be considered in this category. In some hospitals it may include nursing supervisors and assistant administrators for ambulatory care. In other systems, it may include the director of nursing and the hospital administrator. It is vitally important for the program planner to assess the individual system. The goal is to identify those administrative persons who will oversee and approve the program plans. The administrative personnel with the power to make decisions about triage implementation must be identified.

How Involved

Administration must approve the triage program plan. While it does not have the authority over the determination of client assessment criteria, it does determine important factors such as space renovation, staffing increases, and chart revisions. It is vitally important that the program planner develop a triage program proposal to present to administration. This proposal is detailed in Chapter 8.

Hospital administrations *must fully* support the triage program or the system will fail. Consider, for example, staffing: if administration supports the triage system but refuses to permit a staffing increase, it is impossible for the system to effectively function. *Do not* undertake triage program implementation if administration is *not* behind the project.

Anticipated Resistance Factors

Administrators are most likely to be in favor of the concept but opposed to items that mean more expense or involve more personnel. The program planner should anticipate a healthy struggle in trying to reduce the administration resistance. The program proposal should be a facilitative tool. It is important to remember that in any negotiations, both sides must be prepared to give and take.

The program planner may be required to negotiate for implementation of the program on a six-month trial basis. There are two major points that administration must agree to during the trial period. These are increased staffing to implement the system and temporary space in which to operate the program. The success of the trial program will justify inclusion of these changes on a permanent basis. The program planner should try to anticipate potential resistance factors and identify appropriate negotiation strategies prior to meeting with administration.

Anticipated Educational Needs

The administrators require specific and detailed program plans in order to approve the system. The best method to do this is through the proposal that is detailed in Chapter 8.

Once the triage system is implemented, the program planner should provide continual evaluation information regarding the system's functioning, and client satisfaction.

Extent of Planning and Implementation Involvement

This varies depending on the particular institution. The facility and client record renovations necessitate direct administrative involvement. While it is vital that administration support staff education and provide release time for this to occur, administration is not actively involved in the actual program plans or education.

LABORATORY AND X-RAY DEPARTMENTS

How Involved

These departments are involved to the extent that client procedures are ordered by the triage nurse. The program planner must carefully work with the department heads in each of these areas to determine criteria for procedure ordering.

Anticipated Resistance Factors

Resistance may occur if the department heads are not consulted as the program is being planned, or if the triage nurses are careless in the procedure orders.

Anticipated Educational Needs

The program planner must work with the department heads to inform staff members of the new program. Information should include the procedure orders that will be implemented once triage is operational.

Extent of Planning and Implementation Involvement

The department heads from radiology and the laboratory should participate in the triage planning and education of the nurses. The radiologist should work with the emergency department physician coordinator and the program planner to determine what x-rays should be ordered and the criteria for ordering these x-rays. Likewise, the laboratory director should assist in determining the scope of appropriate laboratory testing. These department consultants should also be involved in the evaluation of these aspects of the program. Both of these program consultants should be directly involved in the nurse education program by presenting the information that interfaces with their respective departments.

AMBULANCE AND EMERGENCY SQUAD PERSONNEL

How Involved

These individuals bring clients into the emergency department. The program planner must determine which "stretcher" clients are to be evaluated in the triage center and which should be sent directly to the "back." Ambulance and squad personnel need to be informed of the new system and their role in entering clients into the triage process.

Anticipated Resistance Factors

If this group is adequately informed, no resistance factors are anticipated.

Anticipated Educational Needs

The program planner should meet with these groups to inform them of the scope of the program, the system functioning, and their role in accessing the new system. Specifically, they must know the parameters for delivering clients to either the triage system or to the "back."

Extent of Planning and Implementation Involvement

None.

How Involved

Obviously, this group is most directly involved in the triage process as care recipients.

Anticipated Resistance Factors

Resistance results from lack of information about what is happening and why. Education about the new system is vital.

Anticipated Educational Needs

The public needs a great deal of information about the new triage program and how it operates. The program planner should plan media coverage and public education prior to the initiation of the triage program. Once the public is informed, they generally support the system. Clients perceive that the new system provides more prompt assessment and continuing re-evaluation. It is also reassuring for the public to realize that immediate physician care is provided when warranted.

Table 7-1
Summary of Who's Who and Their
Involvement in the Triage Process

Who's Who	Directly Involved in Program Planning	Directly Involved in Program Implementation
Nursing Staff		
Registered Nurses	Yes	Yes
Licensed Practical or		
Vocational Nurses	No	Limited
Physician Staff		
Permanent Emergency Department		
Physician Staff	Yes	Limited
House Staff	No	Limited
Community Physicians	No	Limited
Other Emergency Department Staff		
Ancillary Staff	No	Yes
Ward Clerks	Limited	No
Hospital Administration	Yes	Limited
Ambulance and Squad Personnel	No	Yes
The Public	No	Yes

Extent of Planning and Implementation Involvement

Public evaluation of the system's operation is very important to both the staff and administration.

SUMMARY

The list of *who's who* is lengthy, but the characteristics and needs of each group are important to anticipate. Table 7-1 summarizes these groups and the involvement of each. The program planner has a complex project to implement and needs the understanding and support of all involved persons. Each program planner must assess the individual system and add to this list. For each addition, the four areas of consideration must be applied and evaluated.

Planning the Triage System

Chapter 8

The initial step in planning the triage system is to identify the type and scope of system needed. The best method to evaluate this is to ask a series of questions about the emergency department's current client flow system and the scope of services offered. From these questions, the program planner must attempt to visualize the changes necessary to implement triage. The planner must then formalize these revisions into a triage program proposal that is the clear statement about the proposed changes in the current system.

THE QUESTIONS

There are three types of data that must be collected. These are identification of information about the current system's functioning, identification of potential change requirements, and identification of the significant persons involved in or affected by the triage process.

Information Data

1. How many clients are seen in your emergency department?
    a.   How many from 7:00 a.m. to 3:00 p.m.?

    b.   How many from 3:00 p.m. to 11:00 p.m.?

    c.   How many from 11:00 p.m. to 7:00 a.m.?

2. Triage is necessary when the number of clients coming into the emergency department exceeds the department's ability to provide immediate care. Based upon the numbers stated above, indicate the times you anticipate needing triage:
    7:00 a.m.–3:00 p.m. _____
    3:00 a.m.–11:00 p.m. _____
    11:00 p.m.–7:00 a.m. _____
    (also consider split combinations such as 11:00 a.m.—1:00 p.m.)

3. During peak hours how many clients on an average do you see during a given hour?

    Remember that it will take an average of three to five minutes for the triage nurse to initially assess each client. Therefore, if you are seeing more than 15 to 20 clients during each hour, you will probably need more than one triage nurse. Likewise, if your department sees fewer than 10 clients per hour, one triage nurse and one ancillary staff will most likely be able to both triage and reassess waiting clients.

Areas Requiring Change

1. What do you anticipate the triage staffing needs to be?

	7:00 am–3:00 pm	11:00 pm–3:00 pm	11:00 pm–7:00 am
Number of Triage Nurses			
Number of Float Nurses			
Number of Ancillary Staff			

2. How many additional staff do you require to implement the triage system?

   What is the cost of this staffing increase?

3. What do you expect the scope of the triage process to include?

   Check as many as are appropriate:
   a. Initial assessment_____
   b. Vital signs (TPR, BP)_____
   c. First aid_____
   d. X-ray ordering (scope of)_____
   e. Laboratory ordering (scope of)_____
   f. Sending clients to other departments or to physician offices_____
   g. Reassessments at prescribed intervals_____

4. What will your system look like? Develop a blueprint with boxes and arrows similar to Figure 4-1 in Chapter 4 that details the flow of clients through your system; whom they will see; and the extent of their assessment and reassessment.

5. If clients are sent to other locations, determine what those locations are, and the necessary arrangements that must be made. List potential referral sites:

    a.

    b.

    c.

    d.

    e.

    f.

    g.

6. What structural renovations are necessary to implement a comprehensive triage center?

    Discuss the temporary operation facilities that will be used while the permanent renovations are being negotiated:

    (It is vital for the program planner to have thought through all structural needs both temporary and permanent prior to presenting the triage proposal to administration.)

7. Is there adequate charting space on your current emergency department client record for the initial triage assessment and reassessment notes?

   If not, how do you plan to document the triage note?

   (It is *not* recommended that a separate sheet of paper be used unless there is a commitment by the emergency department staff and medical records that this separate sheet *will* become part of the client's permanent emergency department record.)
   Will a revision of the chart be necessary?
   If so, what are the anticipated changes?

8. Once the triage system is operational, how will its efficiency and effectiveness be monitored?

What type of ongoing system evaluation do you plan to use (see Chapter 5)?

People Data

1. In your system's "who's who" who will be affected by the triage system:
    a. In the emergency department?

    b. In the hospital?

    c. In the community?

2. Whom do you envision assisting with the triage program planning?
   a. Who will develop the proposal for administration?

   b. Who will work to finalize the protocols appropriate for your institution?

   c. Who will the physician contact be?

   d. Who are the necessary persons in administration to approve the system?

   e. Who will assume the responsibility for staff education? General education about the proposed triage program? Specific education for the RNs preparing them to be triage agents?

3. How do you plan to educate the public about the new triage program?

THE PROPOSAL

This is a formal document that should be developed to present to administration. This document presents objective data detailing the purpose of your triage system; the plan to be implemented; and the method of evaluating the effectiveness of the system.

The following is a detailed outline for the triage program proposal.

The Introduction

This should include a statement as to the reason this proposal is being submitted. The introduction should include statistics about:

1. The number of clients that are processed through your department on yearly, monthly, weekly, daily, and hourly basis. This should also provide general comments about the types of clients seen.

2. Peak utilization hours.

3. Waiting times for clients during these peak periods.

4. Incident reports resulting from untoward client changes while waiting in the lobby.

5. Client complaints. Detail client complaints about not being seen soon enough or having to wait too long. Use these complaints as part of the justification for the triage system.

Philosophy and Objectives of the Triage System

First, there should be a brief summary of the hospital's philosophy and specifically the philosophy of the emergency department.

Emphasis of those points that discuss quality client care and prompt attention to client needs lends credence to the proposed system.

Second, there should be an introduction to the concept of triage, its history, its objectives, and its effectiveness.

This section of the proposal should link the hospital's philosophy with the proposed triage plans. Specifically, there should be a discussion about how this triage system will promote and fulfill the objectives of the individual hospital.

Benefits of the System

Use the presented statistical data from the introduction to discuss the weaknesses in the current system. Then propose how you anticipate the triage system will, in fact, provide better client care. In select cases, triage may not reduce the overall client time in the emergency department, but it will:

1. Expedite client care through immediate assessment by the triage person.
2. Provide the opportunity to develop a selected client data base.
3. Ensure the establishment of care priorities according to the acuteness of the condition.
4. Decrease client delays by initiating diagnostic procedures.
5. Provide continuous reassessment of the individuals waiting for treatment.
6. Provide the opportunity to identify selected client or family health learning needs.
7. Function as a screening area for individuals needing information.
8. Function as a referral site for selected clients not requiring emergency care.
9. Relieve congestion in critical treatment areas and improve traffic flow by utilization of a variety of health care resources.
10. Assist in effective utilization of space and personnel through the assignment of clients to designated treatment areas.
11. Promote rapport through immediate demonstration of concern for emergency department client problems (immediately upon arrival in the emergency department).
12. Have built-in mechanisms for continued system evaluation.

13. Decrease anxiety levels of client and family by producing immediate and ongoing assessment while the client is waiting for medical care.

14. Improve public relations by providing initial and continued client care "in the lobby."

System Description

Develop the blueprint for the triage system in your institution. Incorporate the significant data from the "questions" segment of this chapter. The system description should address the major points of a comprehensive triage system. Summarized from Chapter 4, these are:

1. Description of how clients will move through the system
2. Triage staffing
3. Protocols for system functioning
4. The client encounter
5. The categorization of clients
6. Chart considerations
7. Reassessment guidelines
8. Triage system space

While this section of the proposal may be the most difficult to develop, it is indeed the blueprint that you will use to implement a triage system in your facility. Take your time, develop it well.

System Monitoring

Discuss the plans for the ongoing evaluation of the following:

1. Efficiency of initial client assessment
2. Accurate categorization of clients
3. Adequacy of documentation
4. Correct x-ray and laboratory ordering
5. Adequacy of client reassessments
6. Overall client time in emergency department
7. Number and type of incident reports related to clients waiting in lobby
8. Overall client waiting time in lobby
9. Number and type of client complaints due to lobby waiting
10. Staff satisfaction (nurse, M.D., ancillary)

Staff Requirements

Discuss the changes in staffing requirements necessary for implementation of the comprehensive triage system. The justification for the increase in RNs and ancillary workers should be derived from data collected under the "questions" in this chapter.

It is vitally important to emphasize that the triage proposal *cannot* be implemented if staffing is inadequate. Administration must value the proposed program to the extent that it "protects" the staffing of the triage center, and does not allow staff members to be pulled from that center to assist with client care in the "back." This is a very important point and must be very clearly negotiated.

Educational Requirements

It is important to identify those individuals who will require education prior to triage implementation. Review the educational needs for each group listed in the "who's who" section of Chapter 7 and develop your system's educational profile.

The program planner should develop a specific statement referring to the education required for the registered nurses who must perform triage. The requirements for this education are discussed in detail in Chapter 12. It is important for administration to know who must be educated, what they will be taught and why, and how much time the education will take.

Client Assessment Criteria

The administration should be informed about the protocol concept, criteria for categorizing, and system utilization of the established protocols. Several examples of the protocols should be included in the proposal.

Time Table

The last part of the proposal should include a realistic time frame for planning and implementing the proposed system. The time will vary from 2 months to 18 months depending upon how "unfrozen" your current system is. Analyze the situation and try to determine realistic target dates.

The proposal will clearly describe the need for triage and will provide the specific details of how to implement the triage system in your hospital. The triage proposal is the blueprint for the anticipated system.

Unfreezing

Chapter 9

To unfreeze means to unsettle, to break up current ways of thinking and acting. The change agent works to bring new information that will encourage system members to reconsider the current methods of operation. During the stage of unfreezing, that change agent or program planner introduces information about current operations as well as new ideas that will change and improve the manner in which services are offered.

PROCESS GUIDELINES

Following are several guidelines for the program planner regarding the process of unfreezing:

1. Don't start before you are ready: This very simple statement is similar to "don't leap before you look." The results of premature action could mean suicide. Prepare basic thoughts and plans before you start meeting with personnel. Know what the overall program will look like. Antici-

pate system members' concerns and be prepared to clarify specific points.

2. Keep an open mind: You will be only as successful as system members allow you to be. Be open to their thoughts and ideas. System members must feel that they are part of the program and that they are permitted to participate in the program planning.

3. Learn to work with system members: Capitalize on their enthusiasm. Be prepared to delegate work to members within the system. Good areas for personnel to concentrate work are:
   a. developing protocols that may deviate from those presented in this text
   b. planning for paramedic or public education

Items not to delegate include:
   a. the proposal to administration
   b. negotiations regarding structural or chart revisions
   c. physician education

Each of these items carries a potential for total system failure and, thus, should be handled carefully by the program planner.

4. Be prepared to negotiate: Negotiations are the key to system implementation. As the plans for the triage program are unveiled, resistance points will be quickly identified. Do not attack those points, but gather data about the rationale for the resistance. Use that information and decide which points can be built into the current proposal and which points should be disregarded. Then meet repeatedly with those individuals or groups offering the resistance until acceptable compromises are reached.

During the period of unfreezing, the program planner must remain alert to personnel who continually appear to block the unfreezing attempts. These persons must be assessed for power status and influence in the system. If the blocking is done by persons with much system power, then the potential for triage implementation must be reevaluated.

Triage can be implemented only if system members want it to be implemented. The program planner must provide adequate support and education to facilitate this project. The program planner must unfreeze current thinking and methods of operation.

PROCEDURAL GUIDELINES

The following steps may be used to assist unfreezing:

1. Meet with significant emergency department nurses to share the triage concept and collect their ideas about a system plan for your facility.

2. Prepare the basic plan, develop the who's who, and draft the program proposal. The program planner should begin with a basic program already in mind.

3. Meet with administration. Share information regarding the statistics (as indicated in Chapter 8) of current client numbers seen in the emergency department and current flow problems. It may take several meetings with administration to verify the need for a change in client processing. Do not present the proposal at this point. Request permission to continue to explore the concept and to present a proposal at a later date.

4. Meet with the physician director of the emergency department. As with administration, share your ideas and overall conceptual plan. Clarify that you will share details as they are developed. Also communicate that as the medical components of the system are developed, consultation with the physician director will be sought.

5. Meet with the staff—ail staff members, RNs, LPNs, or LVNs, ancillary workers, and ward clerks. Present the concept of triage and the overall plan that you have in mind. Include in the discussion the role envisioned by each staff member and the differences in role from the current mode of operations. Then sit back and listen to their comments. Don't become defensive; just collect their ideas and their concerns. Your job is to clarify their questions and to gather their ideas.

    From this meeting the program planner should be able to identify points of resistance and areas where unfreezing education is needed. This information should provide content for subsequent meetings with the staff. Following the initial meeting, it may be most beneficial to meet with subsystem staff groups or even individuals to clarify or negotiate specific program plans. It is at this point that the program planner should begin to work with a variety of staff members, involving them in the more detailed plans for the triage program.

    It is vitally important to talk up the concept and to be alert to staff concerns. The program planner can then work specifically to clarify the concerns that have been expressed.

6. Meet with the physician director to present the triage proposal. It is important to meet with the physician prior to presenting the actual proposal to administration. The program plans are most likely to succeed if the program planner and the physician in charge agree on the program's scope and plans. If there are wide differences between the physician in charge and the program planner, those differences must be negotiated prior to going to administration.

7. Present the proposal to administration. This should first be done informally with those administrative persons who are most directly involved with the delivery of emergency services. Following their approval and endorsement, work with those administrative persons to present the proposal to higher level administration. While support for the entire proposal is desirable, support for certain segments is absolutely mandatory.

    These are:
    a. Staffing requirements:
        1. support for adequate staffing
        2. a promise that staff will not be pulled from the triage system.
    b. Staff education: support for the formal education for the RN staff in preparation for system implementation.
    c. Space allocation: appropriate renovations to accommodate the triage program. This may follow a six-month program implementation pilot.

8. Communicate the proposed time table to all staff members. This is done following the formal approval of the proposal. All staff members should be aware of the time and scope outline for the program implementation.

9. Elicit planning and implementation assistance from staff members. This is the time for staff members to plan education programs for community physicians, paramedics, and the public; to finalize protocols and gain physician approval; and to plan for the specific space and client record changes.

SUMMARY

Systems will unfreeze at different levels and speeds depending upon the skill of the program planner. The quality of the program proposal and the objective education of the staff members about the need to change will most likely influence the speed at which a system is unfrozen. Unfreezing is difficult. To succeed, there must be a great deal of commitment and hard work by the program planner.

Unfreezing is the time for planning implementation of the triage system. Certainly the first step of that is planning the system, and communicating the plan to all concerned. Once that is done and everyone at all levels of operation is in agreement that this is the program to use, the system has been adequately unfrozen and is ready to move.

Moving

Chapter 10

Moving is the period of triage system implementation. This includes the specific preparations leading up to the day of implementation as well as the program's actual implementation. Everything that occurs in this phase should be in preparation for the first day of the program implementation. All triage plans have been detailed, and all systems are in support of the project.

There are many personnel groups needing specific education prior to the system's implementation. These groups were referred to in Chapter 7, "Who's Who in System Assessment". These groups will again be briefly discussed to highlight the specific implementation education needs prior to starting triage. The education discussed at this point deals with program details and the specific implementation mechanics. In no way does this discussion replace the need for the "unfreezing" education as described in Chapter 7.

PEOPLE PREPARATION

Registered Nurses

The details of the registered nurse's education are extensive. These details are discussed in Chapter 12.

Licensed Practical Nurses and Ancillary Workers

Both these groups need to know the specific details and mechanics of the program. There should be one or more meeting times scheduled to provide the details and allow for questions and clarification. The best method to provide the details is to talk through the triage system, including a discussion of how decisions are made, the rationale for categorization and rechecks, and the specific responsibilties of each to the system.

The following outline may be helpful in organizing educational details:

The Triage System Blueprint

1. The plan for the system
2. How clients will move through the system
3. Categorization and the use of protocols
4. The recheck process
5. X-ray and laboratory ordering
6. The use of green dots
7. The routing of the client record

Personnel

Discussion of various types of personnel to be used in the system and the roles of each.

1. Triage nurse
2. Float nurse
3. Ancillary workers

System Feedback

Discuss the process by which these personnel can provide feedback about the system's functioning and areas of concern. The specifics regarding this area will be detailed later in this chapter.

Permanent Emergency Department Physician Staff and House Staff

Meet with these groups about two days prior to the system implementation. With the medical directors, present the specifics of the program and how the system will affect client care.

When meeting with these physicians, the following points are important:

The Triage System Blueprint

1. Discuss how clients will move through the system.

2. Share specific information about what the triage and float nurses will do. Include examples showing how protocols will be used as guidelines. Discuss criteria for ordering x-ray and laboratory work. Discuss how first aid techniques will be applied.

3. Discuss types of categories, the rationale for categorization, and the color coding system.

4. Discuss the recheck system.

5. Emphasize that the total triage time will take two to five minutes and that clients requiring immediate physician care will not be detained in triage.

6. Prepare physicians for the type of record documentation by the triage and float nurses.

System Feedback

Physician feedback is helpful in keeping the triage system in focus of the department needs. Plans should be made to have an ongoing feedback system that discusses the strengths and weaknesses of the triage program.

Community Physicians

The program planner or a designated alternate should plan to attend a medical staff meeting with the emergency department's medical director just prior to the system implementation. At this time, the community physicians should be given the following information:

1. Details of the proposed system

2. How the system will help their clients

3. How they may access the triage system to assist with the processing of their clients

4. How the triage system is planned to assist the processing of all clients

5. How they can provide feedback about system functioning and suggestions for improvement

Ambulance and Emergency Squad Personnel

It is vitally important that these persons be informed about the new triage program. This can be effectively handled through a special meeting with the triage planner. Another option is for the designated personnel to visit the various ambulance or squad stations to disseminate the information. Either way, the educational program should occur about two weeks prior to the system implementation. Twenty-four hours before triage begins, a memo should be sent to all ambulance and emergency squad stations reminding them of the changes in operating procedure.

Overview of System Blueprint

1. Why the system is being developed and what it will accomplish

2. Client flow through the system

3. Role of the triage system personnel

4. Overview of the categorization system

Ambulance and Squad Interface with Triage System

1. Description of what type of clients the ambulance and squad personnel should escort directly to the emergency treatment center and what kind of clients should be brought through the triage system

2. Procedures for accepting clients from squad personnel

3. Communication procedures whereby the triage center will be informed about clients being brought by emergency squads and ambulances

4. If triage will not be operational 24 hours per day, a delineation of what the EMTs and paramedics are to do with clients during the shutdown periods

Ward Clerks and Medical Record Personnel

Arrange a meeting with these persons to provide program details and clarify areas of confusion. Specifically cover the following:

Overview of System Blueprint

1. Why the system is being developed and what it will accomplish
2. The process by which clients will be processed through the system
3. The role of the triage nurse, float nurse, and ancillary personnel
4. The process of categorization and the use of different colored arm bands

The Interface of Ward Clerks and Medical Record Personnel with the Triage System

1. Discuss the flow of the chart through the triage system.
2. Discuss the initiation of laboratory and x-ray requisitions.
3. Discuss the role of the ward clerk when new emergency department clients come to the desk for assistance.
4. If triage is not operational 24 hours per day, discuss the client flow system that will be used during system shutdown hours.

X-Ray and Laboratory Personnel

Approximately three or four days prior to the initiation of the triage system, meet with these groups separately to inform them about the new program and how it will affect them. It will be helpful to have the director of the respective departments present to support the changes and give additional clarification. Remember that the department directors should have been involved in the program planning.

The meeting should cover the following points:

1. Overview of the triage system including the purpose and process
2. Discussion of how triage will affect these departments. Specifically, discuss how requisitions will be initiated and

how the various departments should handle the processing of these clients and the results of the specific studies.

Community Education

Approximately one month prior to initiating the program, contact the television and major newspaper representatives in the community. If there are several smaller community newspapers, these may also be contacted. Convey to these persons your wish to provide community education about the triage program one to two days before the program is actually started. Ask these representatives to assist in distributing appropriate information. If your hospital has a public relations or development department, the staff should be able to be of assistance in making the appropriate contacts.

The news media will need information about the following areas:

1. Why the triage system is being initiated. Share statistics about the increased use of the department and how triage will better handle the clients using the department.

2. What the new system will mean for clients. Discuss the differences in client processing:
   a. Emphasize how the new system will offer quick, more comprehensive evaluation of clients as they enter the emergency department.
   b. Discuss the initiation of first aid treatment, x-rays, and laboratory assessment.
   c. Emphasize how those clients requiring immediate care will be sorted out to receive that care.
   d. Discuss the recheck procedures for those clients who must wait for treatment.

DEPARTMENT PREPARATION

Simultaneously with the education of specific personnel groups as just described, the program planner must also prepare the department for the first day of system operation. The major preparations for the system include:

Facility Preparation

The triage space must be prepared (whether this is temporary or permanent) approximately two weeks prior to the initiation of the system. Supplies must be adequate to provide appropriate first aid, and to make initial client assessments including temperature, blood

Table 10-1
Triage Center Supply List

Ice	Disposable diapers	Dextrostix
Ice bags	Washcloths	Lancets
Arm and leg splints	Towels	Antipyretics
Arm slings	Cottonballs	Thermometers
4 × 4s	Eye patches	Sphygmomanometer
Wound cleansing supplies	Tongue blades	Scales
Ace bandages	Emesis basins	Otoscope
Tape	Kleenex	Vision screening chart
Kerlix	Kling	Alcohol swabs
Blood collection supplies		

pressure, and weight. A detailed triage supply list is found in Table 10-1. The triage facility must also have a telephone and an intercom to elicit personnel assistance from the major emergency treatment rooms. Do not permit triage to begin unless the physical facility is ready.

Dry Run

Twenty-four hours prior to the initiation of the new triage program, plan a dry run. Meet with significant personnel to clarify last minute concerns staff may have. Orient the triage nurses to the triage facility and talk through the triage process. Finally, walk through the system to clarify the procedural operations.

The Day of Triage Implementation

The program planner must work as an overseer on the first day of triaging. As clients enter the system there will probably be confusion and an initial slowdown in client processing. The program planner and the float nurse must assist in the initial screening of clients. The first day and most likely the entire first week will make triage appear to be slowing down the process of registering and assessing clients. The system is new and it will take a few days to "get the bugs out." The program planner must anticipate a little confusion and act as a buffer so that staff members and physicians do not get frustrated.

The triage nurses will probably be slow. They must be reminded of the amount of interview time they are using, and the number and types of clients waiting for their assessment. During the first few days of the system's operation, it is also important for the program planner to assist the triage nurse in maintaining a perspective of the total triage operation. The triage nurse must learn to interview and categorize clients while simultaneously assessing the overall triage demands.

It is vitally important that the triage system succeed during the first week. The program planner should prepare to add additional triage nurses or float nurses to maintain a smooth operation. It is also imperative for the program planner to be physically present in the triage facility as much as possible during the first week. The primary responsibility of the program planner during this period is to troubleshoot any system disturbances.

The program planner should arrange a series of conferences to evaluate and ultimately facilitate the mechanics of the system's functioning. The first conference should be with the appropriate workers at the end of each shift. This session should simply be a time of debriefing and sharing about how the first day went. Similar sessions should be held at the end of the first week. The only system evaluation at this time should be to evaluate directly the mechanics of the system's functioning.

The System in Operation

At some given point about a week into the system's operation, the triage process will stabilize. This information should be communicated to all those who are doing their jobs "effectively" and "efficiently." Suddenly, things will begin to click. It is at this point that the program planner must turn attentions to the system's refreezing process. The triage system evaluation must move from evaluation of the mechanics to evaluation of the effectiveness of the system. This will include evaluation by personnel in the sub- and suprasystems. This evaluation and other components of refreezing are discussed in detail in Chapter 5 and the next chapter.

Refreezing

Chapter 11

Refreezing as described in Chapter 1 is the process of reestablishing the system at a higher level of functioning. The refreezing process will determine the system's ability to maintain the new level of operation. The consequences of the change need to be evaluated at each level of the system as integration of that change is contingent upon the payoffs, positive reinforcement, and congruence with the existing value orientation.

As part of the evaluation process, the satisfaction of the system personnel needs to be assessed. Anticipated payoffs that have importance for triage personnel, emergency department personnel, and administrative personnel include:

1. Consistent quality in client assessments and reassessments

2. High quality triage: accurate triage decisions and referrals

3. Greater efficiency in the triage process

4. Decreased waiting time for clients with serious or potentially serious problems

5. Decreased confusion and congestion within the emergency department

6.   Decreased stress levels of the triage agents due to staffing patterns

7.   Increased client and community satisfaction

8.   Decreased emergency department time for clients requiring selected x-ray and laboratory evaluation

9.   Decreased number of clients leaving against medical advice

10. Increased information about clients waiting to be seen

11. Decreased number of incident reports generated from problems occurring in the lobby

Chapter 5 discusses evaluation of the triage system functioning. The data obtained from the evaluation process can be utilized during this refreezing phase as indicators of whether the payoffs are, in fact, occurring. Multiple sources of data are available: triage personnel, emergency department personnel, clients, and client care records. Table 11-1 indicates which component(s) of the evaluation process as described in Chapter 5 will provide data pertinent to the anticipated payoffs.

Positive reinforcement for change can be internal or external. In order for internal positive reinforcement to occur, the triage personnel must be adequately prepared for their function. Inadequate preparation will cause personnel stress, create snags in the flow of the system, and eventually disillusion the persons working in and with the system. The triage personnel need to feel confident about and competent in the performance of their functions. Evaluation data from nursing and medical personnel about client assessments and triage decisions will indicate the strengths and pitfalls of the triage education program. This information should be directed back into the preparation process with incorporation of necessary revisions.

Positive reinforcement can also come from external sources or impinging systems. Feedback from triage personnel, other emergency department personnel, clients, and administrative personnel can provide information about the system's functioning and perceived successes. Administration must demonstrate support of the triage program by enforcing staffing and construction commitments. A continued commitment from administration not to "pull" staff is necessary to ensure sufficient and appropriate personnel to work the system. This tangible reinforcer is critical to the viability of the system. The structural evaluation described in Chapter 5 provides information regarding the success of staffing and staffing patterns.

Administration also needs positive reinforcement about the

Table 11-1

Sources of Data for Evaluation of Payoffs

Payoff	Evaluation Component		
	Structure	Process	Outcome
Consistent quality in client assessments and reassessments.			X
High quality triage: accurate triage decisions and referrals.			X
Greater efficiency in the triage process.		X	
Decreased waiting time for clients with serious or potentially serious problems.		X	X
Decreased confusion and congestion in the emergency department.		X	X
Decreased stress of triage agents due to staffing patterns.	X		
Increased client and community satisfaction.		X	X
Decreased emergency department time for clients requiring selected x-ray and laboratory evaluation.		X	
Decreased number of clients leaving against medical advice.		X	
Increased information about clients waiting to be seen.	X		X
Decreased number of incident reports generated from problems occurring in the lobby.		X	

change. Administrative personnel need to know that the new system is perceived as valuable and effective by staff members and clients.

The data from the process and outcome evaluations as described in Chapter 5 can act as positive reinforcers at all levels regarding the effective and efficient functioning of the new system.

Congruence with existing value orientation is necessary for integration of the system change. Values about the triage system should be similar for those persons who were actively involved in the unfreezing and moving phases of the change process. During the unfreezing process, values about the system, its purpose, and goals were clarified and evaluated. This resulted in individuals acting on the chosen values, which occurred during the moving phase. Some value changes and acquisitions may have had to occur during this process. Continued input from and discussion with personnel will enable the program planner to monitor the commitment to and integration of those values. This is an opportunity to assist individuals in value affirmation supporting the change. Recognition of the payoffs and cognizance of reinforcers strengthen the value choices. Those values that are important to individuals will be acted on consistently and predictably, thus ensuring the refreezing of the system at the new level.

When new personnel are introduced into the system, they too must achieve value congruence in order to act in a manner that supports the new system. There will always be a need for an ongoing triage education program, which will assist new personnel to acquire information about the triage process, and to affirm and eventually integrate the values necessary for maintenance of a comprehensive and successful program.

REFERENCES

Menke, Edna M. Persistence, change and crisis, in Hall, Joanne and Barbara Weaver, editors: Distributive nursing practice: a systems approach to community health, Philadelphia, 1977: J.B. Lippincott Company, pp. 51–56.

Steele, Shirley M. and Vera M. Harmon. Values clarification in nursing, New York, 1979: Appleton-Century-Crofts.

The Registered Nurse Education Program

Chapter 12

The most specific education required for implementation of the triage program is teaching the RNs *how* to triage. Most experienced emergency department nurses are quite proficient at making quick assessments and "ah-ha's" about what is wrong with any given client. What the program planner or designated educator must do is to "unteach" some of the nurses' current practices and re-educate these nurses to make objective and consistent assessments. This is the primary reason for establishing the protocols in Part 3 of this text.

It is the goal of the project educator to prepare the RNs so that, with any given client, all nurses would make assessments based on the same criteria, and each would assign the same categorization. It is *not* the purpose of the education or the triage process to teach these nurses to diagnose the client's problem. The goal is to assess the client's problem and determine the urgency with which that client must receive physical care.

PROPOSED EDUCATIONAL PROGRAM

Following is a proposed educational program. The program may be condensed if all nurses possess physical assessment skills.

Program Rules

1. Every nurse who will assume the role of triage or float nurse must attend the educational program.
2. Attendance at *all* classes is mandatory.

Program Length

The most important consideration at the completion of the educational program is that the nurse students understand the proposed system and be able to use consistent assessment techniques to similarly triage clients through that system. A 24-hour course divided into eight sessions permits adequate time for student preparation. Remember, the triage system must be able to function the day it opens. There may be persons standing around with skeptical viewpoints. The nurses must operate at 100 percent proficiency. Don't skimp on their educational preparation.

Program Objectives

1. To teach the nurses the specific details of the proposed triage system.
2. To teach nurses to collect consistent subjective and objective data on all clients processed through the triage system.
3. To teach the nurses the criteria and process for ordering appropriate x-ray and laboratory studies.
4. To teach the nurses the appropriate data for client record documentation.
5. To teach the nurses *how* to record the data.
6. To teach the nurses how to screen for selective primary health care needs of the client.

Sample of a Proposed Education Program

Table 12-1 shows a complete and comprehensive program. There is ample time in this program for initial presentations by the instructor and practice sessions for the nurse students. The first two classes are presentations of the proposed triage program and the techniques of subjective data collection. The subsequent classes follow a consistent format. Each class period includes the following:

1. Review of anatomy and physiology of the given system.
2. Review of subjective data to be collected per protocol.
3. Review of objective data appropriate for the given system.
4. Review of examination strategies.
5. Review of appropriate x-ray and laboratory procedures for the given system.
6. Common "green dot" needs associated with the given system.
7. Review of developed protocols for the given system.
8. Case study presentation.
9. Practice session using the case study and protocols.

Table 12-1
Triage Education Program*

Session 1:
  Introduction
  Overview of Triage as a Nursing
   Process
  Legal Considerations
	Session 5:
	  Analysis Continued
	   Genitourinary system
	   Musculoskeletal system

Session 2:
  Client Assessment Overview
  Subjective Data Collection
	Session 6:
	  Analysis Continued
	   Integumentary system
	   Ear, nose, throat regions
	   Visual system

Session 3:
  Introduction to Client Protocols
  Analysis of Specific Systems**
   Respiratory system
   Cardiovascular system
	Session 7:
	  Viewing the Client as a Whole
	  Screening for Abuse
	  Nutritional Screening
	  Primary Care Screening

Session 4:
  Analysis Continued
   Central nervous system
   Gastrointestinal system
   Hematolymphatic system
	Session 8:
	  Putting It All Together
	  Anticipated System Problems
	  Summary

* Each class session lasts three hours.

** Use client protocols and actual emergency department cases for practice sessions.

CLASSROOM NUGGETS

Instructional Format

The most important thing to remember is that the nurse students must have time to practice. They must practice collecting subjective and objective data in a consistent manner in a short period of time. The client protocols should be used over and over to reinforce uniformity in data collection and analysis.

Role play is a good format for class practice. It is easiest to use actual cases allowing one nurse to act as the client and the other as the nurse. If the same case is presented to all practice groups, then at the end of the role play experience, the groups can rejoin to compare write ups and categorization.

Time

In the real triage setting, time is the enemy. The nurse must practice reducing the amount of time it takes to collect and record data without compromising the quality. During the classroom sessions, the nurses must practice reducing the triage time from 15 or 20 minutes to approximately 5 minutes. This takes a great deal of practice, but it is a reality for efficient operation of the triage system.

Documentation

Nurses have traditionally never been taught how to document a succinct but comprehensive client assessment note. Again, practice is the key. These authors have found that nurses in general have a great deal of difficulty recording appropriate data in the minimal space provided. During the practice session, use duplicate copies of the actual emergency department record and instruct the students to record their findings and the categorization on this sample record. The instructor should then collect the sample writings and critique each in order to give feedback to the nurse students. See Table 12-2 for a sample triage note.

Objective Data Collection

While nurses must learn selected physical assessment skills in order to collect objective data, it is important to remember that the triage center is no place to perform a physical examination. Many nurses are tempted to perform a more extensive assessment than is necessary. The classroom instructor should stress that only essential physical assessment data be collected. Of all the assessment skills the nurse may use, observation is still the most vital in the triage center.

Table 12-2
Sample Triage Note

CC.	"I fell off my bike and hurt my arm."
V.S.	T. 98.4 P. 92 R. 18 BP. 132/68
S:	60 minutes ago, riding bicycle, hit rough spot in road, fell onto (L) hand and forearm. Since injury ↑ swelling and discomfort. Unable to flex or extend wrist. Denies other injuries. No known illness, no allergies or current meds.
O:	(L), distal forearm and wrist appear swollen, deformity noted, bilat. = radial pulses, bilat = hand color. Able to move fingers with slight discomfort.
A:	Category II
P:	Splint, ice, arm sling, x-ray (L) wrist and forearm.

Subjective Data Collection

Subjective data collection is most commonly the mechanism by which the nurse determines the severity of the client's condition. The nurse must have a broad understanding of a complete subjective data base and symptom analysis so that selected portions can be extracted for individual clients. Based upon each individual client situation, the nurse must pose pertinent questions to ascertain the nature and urgency of each client's condition. The program planner or classroom instructor should spend sufficient time to evaluate the students' understanding of complete subjective data base collection, incomplete subjective data base collection, and symptom analysis. A reference for these points is June Thompson and Arden Bowers, *Clinical Manual of Health Assessment* (The C. V. Mosby Company, St. Louis, 1980).

Clinical Decision Making

By far the most complex issue in triaging is decision making for client categorization. Refer to Chapter 13 in Part 3 of this text for a detailed discussion of triage as a decision-making process.

The Triage System Protocols

Part 3

Decision Making—
Using the Protocols

Chapter 13

INTRODUCTION TO THE PROTOCOLS

This part of the text contains the protocols that the triage personnel will use to make triage decisions. Triage is a decision-making process. These protocols are mechanisms for facilitating that process.

The protocols are designed to be used as guidelines only and may need adjustments according to individual institution preference. It is anticipated that once the triage personnel become familiar with the content of the protocols, these protocols will be needed only for reference. As part of the education process for triage as described in Chapter 12, the individuals performing triage will have content input and classroom experience using the protocols. It is essential that all triage nurses participate in this education experience and become competent in the use of the protocols.

The protocols are organized into two segments. The first segment is indexed according to major body systems. This segment provides specific guidelines for collection of subjective and objective data pertinent to the designated system. When screening clients, all specified subjective and objective data should be evaluated. The categories (I-IV) for priority of care are delineated based on the client assessment from this protocol outline.

The second segment is indexed according to the major presenting symptom. This segment further details specific signs and symptoms with the appropriate categorization (I-IV) and selected diagnostic studies for each. This segment also assists the triage nurse in recategorizing clients as changes in client condition occur.

Through utilization of these protocols, the triage nurse will be able to:

1. Determine pertinent and subjective data to be gathered.

2. Make a category decision.

3. Determine appropriate diagnostic procedures to be initiated.

4. Make recategorization decisions as needed.

DECISION-MAKING PROCESS

Despite these specific protocol guidelines, which are the tools for the decision-making process, each triage decision depends upon the knowledge and skills of the nurse doing triage. As methodology for decision-making varies greatly from one individual to another, the discussion of triage as a systematic decision process is warranted.

Problem Identification

The first step is identification of the problem. Ultimately, the triage question that must be answered is "how acute is this client?" That decision is based on identification of what is "wrong" with the client.

Data must be gathered and then interpreted in order to define the client problem. The sources of information are multiple. Subjective data are gathered from the client, family, or friends. Objective data are gathered through observation and may also include the techniques of inspection, palpation, percussion, and ascultation. Guidelines for the information needed are outlined in the protocols.

Data gathering alone is not sufficient for problem identification. The information must also be interpreted. Interpretation is essential in identifying the problem. Interpretation of the data involves identification of what is known and what is not known—what further questions need to be asked, what additional observations need to be made. The "symptom" segment of the protocols gives particular direction to this realm.

There are several factors that influence problem identification. Knowledge, skill, past experiences, and situational characteristics influence problem identification through their effect on data gathering and interpretation.

The triage nurse's knowledge helps determine the type of information sought, the sources of information utilized, and the interpretation of the data. Data gathering and interpretation become more precise with increased knowledge about a situation. Individuals with limited knowledge about certain factors may be restricted in identification and interpretation of the problem. More information facilitates more precise data gathering, which results in higher level interpretation.

Skill may influence problem identification in a similar manner. Skill in observation, in assessment techniques, and in interviewing adds important information to data collection. The nurse's level of skill will determine the quality and preciseness of information elicited.

Past experience is a factor that can have either a beneficial or detrimental influence on data collection and interpretation. Past experience is a variable that affects the nurse's perception of or reaction to the triage situation. Past experience can enable an individual to better utilize gathered data. On the other hand, it may cause the triage nurse to jump ahead and make an interpretation without fully assessing the situation.

The characteristics of a situation will affect an individual's data gathering and interpretation. The limited time permitted for triage is an important variable that determines the scope of information gathered. The client's physical state and ability to describe his or her situation will affect the amount and type of information gathered. The physical and psychological state of the triage nurse is a factor. The perceptual field of an individual who is feeling tired, anxious or overwhelmed is narrowed and the information that person is able to receive and process may be limited in amount and scope.

Options and Alternatives

Once the client's problem is assessed, the next step is to identify and analyze the options and alternatives. The identification phase is facilitated by the triage categories that have been established as the options for priority of client care. Additionally, the triage nurse must identify the available care areas, resources, or alternatives.

The second phase involves analysis of each of the options in regard to desirability, probability, and risk. Desirability is defined as an individual's preference for an alternative. This preference is influenced by values and feelings. A new, inexperienced triage nurse might prefer to choose higher priority categories in order to be "safe." However, desirability also has to be assessed for the particular situation, and situation constraints have to be identified. In the emergency department situation, while it would be desirable to have everyone seen immediately, the manpower, space, and time available do not usually allow that.

The probability of the success of each of the options and alternatives is a consideration. Will the option work? Is the category appropriate? These are questions that require a knowledge base and past experience to answer. Both knowledge and past experience have been used to establish criteria for client care categories so usage of these categories should provide a high degree of probability.

The degree of risk is the third consideration when analyzing the options. The risk to the client must be evaluated. What will happen if the client is not cared for immediately? Will this client be "okay" if care is postponed? The benefits of such a decision are also weighed. In the emergency department the primary benefit is that, in deciding priorities, the most seriously ill and injured receive immediate care. The balance of risk and benefit is weighed.

Making the Decision

The importance of each of the three areas of analysis (desirability, probability, degree of risk) varies from person to person and situation to situation. The analyzed pieces may be in conflict or congruence. In any instance, the nurse doing triage acts on the basis of which has higher priority for that situation: desirability, probability, or risk. In the emergency department situation, analysis may show that risk has priority over probability or vice versa. The triage person makes the choice, assigns the client to a care category, and directs the client to a specific care area.

As in data gathering, the factors that influence the decision are knowledge, past experience, time, resources, and other situational characteristics.

Evaluating the Decision

A decision can be evaluated on two levels:

1.   Was the decision good?
2.   What was the outcome?

A good decision does not assure a favorable outcome. A good decision is derived from all phases of the decision-making process. If a decision was made utilizing all the elements of the process in a systematic manner, then the decision was a good one.

However, in dealing with life-threatening injuries or illnesses, the outcome is the basis of evaluation of the triage decision. In an emergency department, the final client outcome cannot always be favorable, but the triage outcome can be evaluated by assessing the following areas:

1. Were the appropriate data gathered?
2. Was the client correctly triaged?
3. Did the client suffer any consequences from waiting?
4. Was the client directed to an appropriate area?

The evaluation of the triage outcome is the basis for the ongoing evaluation of the effectiveness of the entire triage process.

REFERENCES

Baldridge, Patricia B.: The nurse in triage, Nurs. Outlook, 14(11): pp. 46-48, November 1966.

Ford, Jo Ann G., Louise N. Trygstad-Durland, and Bobbie C. Nelms. Applied decision making for nurses, St. Louis, 1979: The C.V. Mosby Company.

Nyberg, Jan: Perception of patient problems in the emergency department, J.E.N., 4(1): pp. 15-19, January/February 1978.

The Protocols

INSTRUCTIONS FOR USING PROTOCOLS

The protocols have all been developed in a consistent format. This format will facilitate their use in a reference situation. Following is a description of the format as well as instructions as to how the flow sheets are to be used.

The reader is reminded that the protocols have been developed as guidelines only. The professional nurse is expected to individualize this information as each client is assessed.

PROTOCOL FORMAT	INSTRUCTIONS FOR USE
1. Major system represented by protocol	The index following these instructions outlines the major systems that have been developed, as well as the contents of that system.

2. Subjective and objective data about the major system or selected components of the major system

After the nurse identifies the appropriate system, or appropriate component of the system (i.e. medical versus trauma), the identified subjective and objective data should be collected.

3. Flow sheets

97 flow sheets representing client complaints have been developed to assist the nurse in correctly assessing and categorizing each client. Data have been clustered so that a client with specific subjective and objective signs will receive the correct priority of care.

The nurse is directed to categorize the client based upon the presence of stated data.

4. Summary categorization sheets

At the end of each major system is a collective list of the complaints listed in that system as well as the appropriate categorization of each.

PROTOCOL INDEX

	TOPIC	PAGE

The Protocols

1. BILIARY
2. CARDIOVASCULAR
3. DENTAL
4. EAR
5. EYE
6. FEVER
7. FLUID AND ELECTROLYTE/ACID BASE
8. GASTROINTESTINAL/ABDOMINAL
9. GENITOURINARY
10. HEMOTOLYMPHATIC
11. INGESTIONS
12. INTEGUMENTARY
13. MOUTH AND THROAT
14. MUSCULOSKELETAL
15. NEUROLOGICAL
16. NOSE AND NASAL
17. PSYCHOLOGICAL STRESS
18. RESPIRATORY
19. TOXIC SUBSTANCES

1
2
3
4
5
6
7
8
9
10
11
12
13
14
15
16
17
18
19

MAJOR SYSTEM: BILIARY

Subjective and Objective Data   **Flow Sheets**

Biliary   Jaundice

Subjective Assessment

1. Describe onset of current problem and pattern of problem since onset.

2. Describe associated symptoms since onset: pain, itching, nausea, vomiting, diarrhea, appetite, etc.

3. Is problem becoming worse or better?

4. History of chronic diseases such as liver disease, gall bladder, alcoholism, hepatitis, others.

5. Have others at home been ill? Anyone else with jaundice?

6. History of recent surgery or blood transfusion.

7. Currently taking any medications?

Objective Assessment

1. General observations of client's overall status (ill appearing? in severe pain?).

2. Observe degree of jaundice.

SUBJECTIVE AND OBJECTIVE DATA
BILIARY

Signs/Symptoms

Category

Client with jaundice
Also appears ill or is having significant pain   --YES→   CATEGORY II

Client with jaundice
Not feeling well   --YES→   CATEGORY III

Client with jaundice
Skin itches, client feeling O.K.   --YES→   CATEGORY IV

1

**JAUNDICE
BILIARY**

Category I	Category II	Category III	Category IV
	Client with jaundice, also appears ill or is having pain	Client with jaundice, not feeling well	Client with jaundice, skin itches Client feeling O.K.

OVERVIEW
BILIARY

MAJOR SYSTEM: **CARDIOVASCULAR**

Subjective and Objective Data

Flow Sheets

Cardiovascular

Chest Pain

Irregular Pulse or PAT

Fast or Slow Pulse or
Pacemaker Malfunction

CARDIOVASCULAR

2

Subjective Assessment

1. History of cardiovascular disease, or congestive heart failure?

2. Describe current feelings—fatigue, nausea, vomiting.

3. Describe changes during past 24 hours.

4. Associated shortness of breath? Dyspnea? Activity related? Known respiratory problems? Cough?

5. Associated chest pain? Quality? Severity? Traveling? Onset? Duration? Treatment for? Describe discomfort in detail. Palpitations?

6. Leg cramps? Swollen legs?

7. Family history of associated cardiovascular disease?

8. Current medications?

9. Other significant medical problems—hypertension; diabetes; known vascular disease.

Objective Assessment

1. Observations:

   General—posturing, appearance of anxiety or fright, note neck vein distension

   Ventilatory effort indicating difficulty or distress

   Skin—note color, moisture, pallor, cyanosis; note color of nail beds and mucous membranes

   Evidence of chest trauma (bruising, wound)

2. Palpate:

   Chest wall for heaving and subcutaneous emphysema

   Skin for moisture and turgor

   Pulses for intensity and quality (carotid, radial, femoral)

3. Auscultate:

   Respiratory—rate, rhythm, depth, lung sounds

   Cardiac—rate, rhythm, quality, extra sounds

SUBJECTIVE AND OBJECTIVE DATA CARDIOVASCULAR

Signs/Symptoms			Category
Known cardiac Now having new cardiovascular symptoms	-or-	Client with chest pain or jaw pain, shortness of breath, moist skin, nausea	--YES→ CATEGORY I
Client with nonradiating chest pain No breathing difficulty or irregular pulse Client does not look ill			--YES→ CATEGORY II
Client with non-radiating chest pain Seems to be respiratory related No cardiovascular symptoms			--YES→ CATEGORY III
Client with pinpoint chest pain Symptoms leading to muscular-skeletal system Client does not appear ill			--YES→ CATEGORY IV

CHEST PAIN
CARDIOVASCULAR

2

Signs/Symptoms		Category
Client with PAT		
-or- Client with irregular pulse Looks ill or has shortness of breath	--YES→	CATEGORY I
Client with known irregular pulse, now not feeling well Denies shortness of breath or chest pain	--YES→	CATEGORY II

IRREGULAR PULSE OR PAT
CARDIOVASCULAR

Signs/Symptoms			Category
Client with malfunctioning pacemaker Appears ill -or- Client with extreme tachycardia or bradycardia Appears ill	--YES→		CATEGORY I
Client with pacemaker—now presenting because of fast, slow or irregular pulse Client does not appear ill	--YES→		CATEGORY II

FAST OR SLOW PULSE OR PACEMAKER MALFUNCTION
CARDIOVASCULAR

2

Category I	Category II	Category III	Category IV
Known cardiac now having new symptoms	Client with nonradiating chest pain, no breathing difficulty	Client with nonradiating chest pain	Client with pinpoint chest pain
Client with chest pain, shortness of breath	Client does not appear ill	Seems to be respiratory related	Symptoms leading to musculoskeletal system
Moist skin and nausea	Client with known irregular pulse—now not feeling well	No cardiac symptoms	Client does not appear ill
Client with PAT	Denies shortness of breath		
Client with irregular pulse	Client with pacemaker—now presenting because of fast, slow or irregular pulse		
Looks ill or has shortness of breath or chest pain	Client does not appear ill		
Client with malfunctioning pacemaker			
Appears ill			
Client with extreme tachycardia or bradycardia			
Appears ill			

**OVERVIEW
CARDIOVASCULAR**

MAJOR SYSTEM: DENTAL

Subjective and Objective Data

Dental

Flow Sheets

Dental Medical

Dental Trauma

3

DENTAL

Subjective Assessment

1. History of trauma? Describe.

2. Toothache
   Describe onset of and characteristics of.

3. History of similar problems in the past?

4. Last time to dentist.

5. Medication allergies.

6. Systemic complaints:

   Fever

   Nausea

   Vomiting

   Sore throat

   Headache

7. Any chance of aspiration of tooth?

Objective Assessment

1. Trauma:

   Observe gingiva for lacerations or contusions

   Observe buccal mucosa and tongue

   Observe teeth for fracture

   Palpate teeth for looseness or instability

   Palpate jaw and facial bones, mandible, TM joints
   for tenderness

2. Medical:

   Observe external jaw for swelling

   Observe internal mouth for redness, swelling,
   obvious pus

   Palpate gum base of involved tooth

   Evaluate for pus

   Palpate cervical lymph nodes

SUBJECTIVE AND OBJECTIVE DATA
DENTAL

Signs/Symptoms		Category
Toothache, fever and swelling Client very uncomfortable -or- Bleeding gums Client uncomfortable	--YES→	CATEGORY III
Localized toothache No fever or swelling	--YES→	CATEGORY IV

DENTAL MEDICAL
DENTAL

Signs/Symptoms				Category
Multiple teeth knocked out Client with obvious mouth and gum injury	-or-	Tooth or teeth knocked out Client has tooth (teeth) for replacement	--YES→	CATEGORY I
Tooth knocked out and facial or jaw tender to palpation	-or-	Tooth, teeth knocked out Bleeding of gum continues	--YES→	CATEGORY II
Tooth knocked out Client requesting evaluation No gum or other mouth injury			--YES→	CATEGORY IV

DENTAL TRAUMA
DENTAL

Category I	Category II	Category III	Category IV
Multiple teeth knocked out Obvious mouth injury	Tooth knocked out Client having facial or jaw pain	Toothache, fever and swelling Client very uncomfortable	Tooth knocked out Client requesting evaluation No other injury
Teeth knocked out Client has teeth for replacement	Active bleeding following tooth knocked out	Bleeding gums Client uncomfortable	Localized toothache

3

**OVERVIEW
DENTAL**

MAJOR SYSTEM: EAR

Subjective and Objective Data	Flow Sheets
Adult Medical	Earache
Pediatric Medical	Ear Drainage
	Hearing Problems
	Tinnitus
Ear Trauma	Foreign Body
	Trauma

EAR

Subjective Assessment

1. Describe details or problem characteristics: onset (slow versus sudden), cause of problem since onset.

2. How does current problem interfere with hearing?

3. Hearing ability prior to current problem onset? Use of hearing aid?

4. Similar problems in the past? Describe.

5. Associated dizziness, ringing in ears, etc.

6. Current medications? Describe.

7. History of previous ear trauma or ear surgery.

8. History of head trauma? Relationship to current symptoms?

Objective Assessment

1. Observe client for posturing, dizziness, or overt signs of discomfort.

2. Observe external ear for lesions, swelling, discoloration, drainage or blood.

3. Observe external canal for foreign bodies, irritation or swelling.

SUBJECTIVE AND OBJECTIVE DATA—ADULT MEDICAL EAR

Subjective Assessment

1. Describe details of—onset and slow versus sudden onset; progression of symptoms.

2. Character of pain or discomfort.

3. Similar problem in past? Describe.

4. Other symptoms, i.e., cold, congestion, sore throat, headache, fever, dizziness.

5. Possibility of puncture of tympanic membrane?

6. How does mother clean ears?

7. Previous ear surgery (tubes)?

8. Any hearing problems?

9. Current medications?

Objective Assessment

1. Observe child—crying, pulling at ears, verbalizes earache.

2. Observe external ears for lesions, swelling, discoloration, drainage, blood.

3. Observe external canal for foreign bodies, wax plugs, irritation or swelling.

4. Observe general discomfort of child—crying or fussy most of the time versus playful.

4

SUBJECTIVE AND OBJECTIVE DATA—PEDIATRIC MEDICAL EAR

Signs/Symptoms

Category

Acute onset earache, may have fever
Uncomfortable
Cold symptoms may accompany

--YES→   CATEGORY III

Minor earache
Chronic problem
No fever

--YES→   CATEGORY IV

EARACHE
EAR

Signs/Symptoms

Signs/Symptoms		Category
Bloody drainage from ears after trauma	--YES→	CATEGORY I
Ear drainage with fever over 101°	--YES→	CATEGORY III
Ear drainage with fever under 101°	--YES→	CATEGORY IV

4

EAR DRAINAGE
EAR

Signs/Symptoms

Category

Acute onset of significant
hearing loss
No other major problems

--YES→

CATEGORY II

Slow onset of hearing loss
Request for evaluation

--YES→

CATEGORY IV

HEARING PROBLEMS
EAR

Signs/Symptoms

Category

Tinnitus with ingestion history of aspirin-containing drugs -or- Tinnitus with vertigo --YES→ CATEGORY II

Tinnitus with fever over 101° --YES→ CATEGORY III

Tinnitus with fever under 101° --YES→ CATEGORY IV

TINNITUS
EAR

4

Subjective Assessment

1. Describe injury in detail.

2. Time since injury? Treatment since injury?

3. Any hearing loss or dizziness associated with injury?

4. Bleeding or drainage from ears since injury?

5. Possibility of puncture of tympanic membrane? Object inserted into ear canal?

6. History of head trauma?

7. Normal status of hearing ability?

Objective Assessment

1. Observe external ear to evaluate extent of injury.

2. Observe bleeding or drainage from ear (if clear drainage present evaluate for sugar content with dextrostix).

SUBJECTIVE AND OBJECTIVE DATA—EAR TRAUMA EAR

Signs/Symptoms

Category

Foreign body—live bug   --YES→   CATEGORY II

Foreign body—stuck in ear
resulting in bleeding
 -or-
Foreign body in ear causing
discomfort   --YES→   CATEGORY III

Foreign body in ear
No discomfort   --YES→   CATEGORY IV

4

**FOREIGN BODY
EAR**

159

4

Signs/Symptoms

		Category
Amputation of external ear	-or-	Bloody drainage from ear following trauma	--YES→	CATEGORY I

Minor or partial tear of external ear	-or-	Hearing problem Acute onset following trauma	-or-	Cold injury— frostbite and pain of external ear	--YES→	CATEGORY II

TRAUMA
EAR

Category I	Category II	Category III	Category IV
Trauma:			
	Amputation external ear		
	Minor or partial tear—external ear		
	Hearing problem—acute onset following trauma		
Medical:			
Bloody drainage following ear trauma			
Bloody drainage from ear	Acute onset hearing loss	Ear drainage Fever	Slow onset hearing loss
	Tinnitus with ingestion history of aspirin-containing drugs	Tinnitus with fever over 101°	Ear drainage No fever
	Tinnitus with vertigo	Foreign body—stuck in ear: bleeding associated	Tinnitus with fever under 101°
	Foreign body Bug in ear	Foreign body in ear causing discomfort	Foreign body in ear No discomfort
	Cold injury to external ear		

4

OVERVIEW
EAR

MAJOR SYSTEM: EYE

Subjective and Objective Data

Flow Sheets

Eye Medical

        Eye Pain

        Eye or Periorbital Infection

        Visual Change

Eye Trauma

        Eye Trauma

5

EYE

Subjective Assessment

1. Describe details of current eye problem—type onset, time since onset, progression of current problem since onset.

2. History of previous eye problems—describe.

3. How is vision affected by current eye problem—blurred vision, light hurts eyes, partial vision, pain, itching, eye drainage, double vision (describe characteristics)?

4. History of allergy?

5. Associated symptoms such as fever, malaise, nausea, vomiting, headache?

6. History of chronic diseases such as diabetes, hypertension, glaucoma?

7. Current medications?

8. Last eye examination? Wear glasses? Vision ability?

Objective Assessment

1. Visual acuity—near vision, distant vision.

2. Observe external eye and surrounding area:
   Periorbial area—swelling, discoloration, bruising

   Lids—swelling, redness, discoloration, sty

   Bulbar conjunctiva—redness

   Lacrimal passage—pus, increased drainage

   Sclera—check presence of blood (sub-conjunctival hemorrhage), discoloration yellowing, increased vascularization (blue tinge normal in newborn)

   Cornea—opacity

   Anterior chamber—opacity, blood (hyphema)

   Pupil/iris—equal, intact, react to light

3. Observe eye function regarding cranial nerves III, IV, VI.

4. Palpate eye area for tenderness

5. Palpate lacrimal passage for pus excretion.

SUBJECTIVE AND OBJECTIVE DATA—EYE MEDICAL EYE

Signs/Symptoms		Category
Sudden severe eye pain No history of trauma One or both eyes	--YES→	CATEGORY II
Stabbing or shooting eye pain—associated with headache Client very uncomfortable -or- Chronic eye pain, increasing in severity Client very uncomfortable	--YES→	CATEGORY III
Vague or minor eye pain	--YES→	CATEGORY IV

5

EYE PAIN
EYE

Signs/Symptoms		Category
Periorbital swelling Client has fever	--YES→	CATEGORY II
Drainage from eye or lacrimal duct Client with fever	-or- Client with sty	--YES→	CATEGORY III
Crusting or matted substance around eyes No fever	--YES→	CATEGORY IV

EYE OR PERIORBITAL INFECTION
EYE

Signs/Symptoms		Category
Sudden decrease in vision, visual acuity, or visual fields Sudden onset diplopia	--YES→	CATEGORY II
Significant diplopia or change in vision, visual acuity or visual fields over past 24 hours	--YES→	CATEGORY III
Gradual change in vision, visual acuity, or visual fields No sudden changes	--YES→	CATEGORY IV

VISUAL CHANGE EYE

Subjective Assessment

1. Describe specific characteristics of injury.

2. Time since injury and first aid treatment?

3. Description of current vision impairment:

   Blurred vision

   Light hurts eyes

   Partial vision

   Pain

   Eye drainage

   Double vision

4. History of previous eye or vision problems?

5. Health of eyes prior to injury—normal vision?

6. History of chronic systemic diseases—describe.

7. Other injuries besides eye injury?

8. Last tetanus injection?

Objective Assessment

1. Visual acuity—near vision, distant vision

2. Observe external eye and surrounding area—note abrasions, laceraction, hematoma, foreign body:

   Periorbital area

   Lids

   Palpebra conjunctiva

   Bulbar conjunctiva

   Lacrimal passage

   Sclera

   Cornea

   Anterior chamber

   Iris/pupil

3. Observe motor function CN III, IV, VI.

4. Gently palpate eye area for tenderness.

   **Do not palpate eye area if sclera or corneal laceration is anticipated.

SUBJECTIVE AND OBJECTIVE DATA—EYE TRAUMA EYE

Signs/Symptoms

Category

Hyphema -or- Puncture wound to globe -or- Chemical substance in eye -or- Direct burn to eye -or- Blurred or decreased vision following trauma --YES→ CATEGORY I

Corneal abrasion -or- Cigarette burn to eye area -or- Foreign body not able to irrigate out --YES→ CATEGORY II

Foreign body irrigated out --YES→ CATEGORY III

Subconjunctival hemorrhage --YES→ CATEGORY IV

5

EYE TRAUMA
EYE

Category I	Category II	Category III	Category IV
Trauma:			
Hyphema	Corneal abrasion	Foreign body irrigated out	Subconjunctival hemorrhage
Puncture wound to globe	Cigarette burn to eye area		
Chemical substance in eye	Foreign body not able to irrigate out		
Direct burn to eye			
Blurred or decreased vision following trauma			
Medical:	Periorbital swelling	Drainage from eye or lacrimal duct	Crusting or matted substance around eyes
	Client has fever	Client with fever	
	Sudden severe eye pain	Client with sty	Vague and minor eye pain
	No history of trauma	Stabbing or shooting eye pains	
	Sudden decrease in vision, visual acuity or visual fields	May be associated with headache	Gradual change in vision, visual acuity or visual fields
	Sudden onset diplopia	Chronic eye pain increasing in severity	No sudden changes
		Significant diplopia or change in vision, visual acuity, or visual fields during past 24 hours	

**OVERVIEW
EYE**

MAJOR SYSTEM: FEVER

Subjective and Objective Data

Fever

Flow Sheets

Fever

6

Objective Assessment

1. Observe client's overall condition for assessment of seriousness of problem.

2. Record temperature.

3. Generally observe client's skin for rashes, lesions, bites, etc.

Subjective Assessment

1. Describe details of current problem—onset, duration, problem course.

2. Other systemic complaints? Night sweats?

3. History of previous colds, congestion, nausea, vomiting, ache, chills, etc?

4. Others at home ill?

5. History of laceration, insect bites, infections or other injuries during past week?

6. History of rashes?

7. History of febrile convulsions?

8. Current medications (ASA, acetaminophen)—last dose: time and amount?

SUBJECTIVE AND OBJECTIVE DATA
FEVER

Signs/Symptoms

Signs/Symptoms		Category
Current temperature 105° or over	--YES→	CATEGORY I
Client presenting with rapid fever onset History of previous febrile seizure -or- Temperature over 104° Client appears ill	--YES→	CATEGORY II
Temperature over 101° Client appears ill	--YES→	CATEGORY III
Temperature over 101° Client appears O.K. -or- Temperature under 101° Client in no distress	--YES→	CATEGORY IV

FEVER

6

Category I	Category II	Category III	Category IV
Current temperature 105° or greater	Client presents with rapid fever onset History of previous febrile seizure	Temperature over 101° Client appears ill	Temperature over 101° Client appears O.K.
	Temperature over 104° Client appears ill		Temperature under 101°

OVERVIEW
FEVER

6

MAJOR SYSTEM: FLUID AND ELECTROLYTE/ACID BASE

Subjective and Objective Data	Flow Sheets
Blood Glucose Imbalance	Blood Glucose Imbalance
Dehydration or Electrolyte Imbalance	Dehydration or Electrolyte Imbalance, Vomiting and Diarrhea
Heat Distress	Heat Distress
Near Drowning	Near Drowning

FLUID AND ELECTROLYTE/ACID BASE

Subjective Assessment

1. History of chronic problem?

2. Current medication for diabetes—state kind of insulin, last dose; if dose has been skipped, why?

3. Concurrent other medical problems or illness or infections?

4. Food intake past 24 hours?

5. Insulin intake past 24 hours?

6. Urine testing at home? Time last dose? Result of that testing?

7. Other current medications?

8. Reason why client thinks current problem exists? Duration of current problem?

9. Detailed history of distress symptoms from the detailed list (see**).

Objective Assessment

1. General observation of client's degree of illness.

2. Assessment of blood sugar screen by dextrostix.

3. Assessment of urine for sugar and acetone (save specimen for further laboratory analysis).

4. Assessment of classical signs from detailed list (see **).

SUBJECTIVE AND OBJECTIVE DATA—BLOOD GLUCOSE IMBALANCE FLUID ELECTROLYTE/ACID BASE

**CLASSIC SIGNS AND SYMPTOMS OF BLOOD GLUCOSE IMBALANCE:

SUBJECTIVE DATA:

polyuria	polyphagia	coma
glucosuria	vomiting	stupor
ketonuria	nausea	drowsiness
thirst	anorexia	listlessness
polydipsia	abdominal pain	weakness
rapid breathing	shortness of breath	chest pain

OBJECTIVE DATA:

coma	orthostatic hypotension	abdominal tenderness
stupor	fruity odor breath	flaccid muscles
poor skin turgor	rapid deep respiration	decreased tendon reflexes
weak rapid pulse	soft eyes	decreased body weight
hypothermia	dilated pupils	

7

Signs/Symptoms		X-Ray Lab	Category
Client may or may not be known diabetic Now appears ill Needs stabilization and further evaluation	--YES→	May or may not do dextrostix and urine analysis	CATEGORY I
Client may or may not be known diabetic No acute distress, but showing multiple signs of blood glucose related problem	--YES→	Dextrostix and urine analysis	CATEGORY II
Known diabetic No distress Needs new prescription of insulin	--YES→	Dextrostix and urine analysis	CATEGORY IV

BLOOD GLUCOSE IMBALANCE
FLUID ELECTROLYTE/ACID BASE

Subjective Assessment

1. Describe onset of problems and course of problem since onset.

2. Describe amount of characteristics of vomiting and diarrhea.

3. History of others in household who have been ill?

4. History of chronic diseases or similar previous episodes of current problem.

5. Current medications?

6. Describe fluid and food intake during past 48 hours.

7. Describe associated symptoms such as abdominal pain, muscle cramps, headache, blurred vision, muscle weakness, muscle twitching, lethargy or confusion.

Objective Assessment

1. Observe general health and strength of client.

2. Vital signs.

3. Note characteristics of dehydration such as dry mucous membranes, sunken eyes, or lack of perspiration.

SUBJECTIVE AND OBJECTIVE DATA—DEHYDRATION OR ELECTROLYTE IMBALANCE FLUID ELECTROLYTE/ACID BASE

7

7

Signs/Symptoms		Category
Client appears ill, states multiple symptoms indicating severe electrolyte imbalance or dehydration	--YES→	CATEGORY I
Client appears ill and dehydrated -or- Extensive vomiting or diarrhea Client very uncomfortable	--YES→	CATEGORY II
Client gives history of extensive vomiting and/or diarrhea Does not appear to be in distress	--YES→	CATEGORY III
Client gives history of vomiting and diarrhea Does not appear ill	--YES→	CATEGORY IV

DEHYDRATION OR ELECTROLYTE IMBALANCE— VOMITING AND DIARRHEA
FLUID ELECTROLYTE/ACID BASE

Subjective Assessment

1. Describe duration of heat exposure.

2. Describe client signs and symptoms.

3. State fluid intake during past several hours.

4. History of chronic diseases?

5. History of similar problem in past.

6 Current medications?

Objective Assessment

1. Evaluation of vital signs; specifically assess client's core body temperature and cardiovascular status.

2. Observe general distress of client.

7

SUBJECTIVE AND OBJECTIVE DATA—HEAT DISTRESS FLUID ELECTROLYTE/ACID BASE

Signs/Symptoms

		Category
History of heat exposure Client appears ill High core body temperature Lack of perspiration	--YES→	CATEGORY I
History of heat exposure Client now feeling much better Minimal increase in core temperature	--YES→	CATEGORY II

HEAT DISTRESS
FLUID ELECTROLYTE/ACID BASE

7

Subjective Assessment

1. Describe specific details of incident.

2. Salt water or fresh water?

3. First aid or oxygen therapy since incident?

Objective Assessment

1. General observation of client—note overall respiratory distress; alertness; signs of agitation; confusion, or distress.

SUBJECTIVE AND OBJECTIVE DATA—NEAR DROWNING FLUID ELECTROLYTE/ACID BASE

Signs/Symptoms		Category
Client showing distress since near drowning incident	--YES→	CATEGORY I
Client history of near drowning First aid at scene Now client appears in no distress	--YES→	CATEGORY II

NEAR DROWNING
FLUID ELECTROLYTE/ACID BASE

Category I	Category II	Category III	Category IV
Electrolyte imbalance Client appears quite ill May show severe dehydration	Electrolyte imbalance Client appears ill and dehydrated	Client gives history of vomiting and diarrhea Not in distress	Client gives history of vomiting and diarrhea Does not appear ill
History of extreme or extended heat exposure High core body temperature Client very ill Lack of perspiration	Extensive vomiting and diarrhea Client uncomfortable	History of heat exposure Client now feeling better Minimal increase in core temperature	Client known diabetic No current problems Requests blood test or new prescription
Near drowning Client showing distress	History of near drowning First aid at scene Client now appears O.K.		
Client may or may not be known diabetic Now appearing ill Needs stabilization and further evaluation	Client may or may not be known diabetic No acute distress, but showing multiple signs of glucose-related problem		

OVERVIEW
FLUID ELECTROLYTE/ACID BASE

MAJOR SYSTEM: GASTROINTESTINAL/ABDOMINAL

Subjective and Objective Data

Gastrointestinal/Abdominal
  Medical

Gastrointestinal/Abdominal
  Trauma

Flow Sheets

Abdominal Pain

Rectal Bleeding, Pain, Itching

Dysphagia

Navel Swelling or Discharge

Abdominal Trauma

8

GASTROINTESTINAL/ABDOMINAL

Subjective Assessment

1. Symptom onset sudden versus gradual?
2. Describe characteristics of symptoms.
3. Interference of symptoms with play, work or activities of daily living?
4. Symptom associated with eating, bowel movements, voiding, menses, weight loss, activity?
5. When was last bowel movement—note characteristics.
6. If *vomiting*—describe frequency, character, amount, associated cramps, weakness, abdominal pains.
7. If *diarrhea*—describe characteristics, frequency, associated cramps, pain, mucous, blood.
8. Past medical history:
   Similar problems—describe?
   Surgeries (i.e., appendectomy, other)?
   Chronic diseases (e.g., sickle cell, diabetes, adrenal problems)?
9. If sudden onset—question possible ingestion.
10. Pinworms (anal itching, pain)?
11. Female—sexually active (refer to subjective questioning in genito-urinary section)?

Objective Assessment

1. General observation:
   Appearance—alert versus listless, lethargic, curled up in pain versus lying flat?
   Color—pale?
   Skin—moist, dry, decreased turgor?
   Eyes—sunken "tired" eyes?
   Gait and posturing during walking?
2. Observe abdomen:
   Symmetry, visible peristalsis?
   Navel swelling or discharge?
3. Observe characteristics and amount of emesis.
4. Abdominal palpation and auscultation should not be performed in triage.

SUBJECTIVE AND OBJECTIVE DATA—GASTROINTESTINAL/ABDOMINAL
MEDICAL
GASTROINTESTINAL/ABDOMINAL

Signs/Symptoms

Signs/Symptoms			Category
Abdominal pain acute onset with vomiting, dehydration or diarrhea	-or-	Severe abdominal pain with hematemesis	--YES→ CATEGORY I
Severe intermittent abdominal pain with bloody rectal mucous with or without vomiting			
Abdominal pain with rectal bleeding (order H&H)	-or-	Client with possible appendicitis May order CBC, U/A, chest x-ray Acute abdominal series X-ray (following pregnancy screen)	--YES→ CATEGORY II
		Abdominal pain, vomiting and diarrhea Minimal dehydration	
Abdominal pain with vomiting and/or diarrhea Not acutely ill appearing	-or-	Abdominal pain Client with active sexual history (order U/A and pregnancy screen) (see genitourinary protocol)	--YES→ CATEGORY III
Vomiting and diarrhea No history of dehydration	-or-	Constipation	--YES→ CATEGORY IV
		Not eating No other problems	
Pain upon urination Urinary frequency (see genitourinary protocol)	-or-	Cramps, menstrual related	

ABDOMINAL PAIN
GASTROINTESTINAL/ABDOMINAL

8

189

8

Signs/Symptoms

Rectal bleeding or prolapse
Large amount bloody or tarry
stool

--YES→ CATEGORY I

Rectal bleeding
Also having abdominal pain
Client appears pale

-or-

Child under age one year with
rectal bleeding, fever, constipation or diarrhea

--YES→ CATEGORY II

Adult with small amount rectal
bleeding, fever, constipation
or diarrhea

--YES→ CATEGORY III

-or-

Rectal pain or itching

--YES→ CATEGORY IV

Constipation

Category

RECTAL BLEEDING, PAIN, ITCHING
GASTROINTESTINAL/ABDOMINAL

Signs/Symptoms		Category
Difficulty swallowing, client having respiratory distress	--YES→	CATEGORY I
Difficulty swallowing with drooling Swollen glands or tonsils -or- Difficulty swallowing Possible foreign body (No respiratory distress)	--YES→	CATEGORY II
Difficulty swallowing No swollen glands or respiratory difficulty	--YES→	CATEGORY III
Difficulty swallowing, sore throat, sinus congestion	--YES→	CATEGORY IV

8

DYSPHAGIA
GASTROINTESTINAL/ABDOMINAL

8

Signs/Symptoms

Navel swelling sudden onset
Associated severe abdominal
pain

--YES→

Category

CATEGORY I

Chronic navel discharge
Client not ill appearing

--YES→

CATEGORY IV

NAVEL SWELLING OR DISCHARGE
GASTROINTESTINAL/ABDOMINAL

Subjective Assessment

1. Specific description of injury—
   if auto accident, did client hit steering
   wheel or was he wearing seat belt?

2. Symptoms of cramping or pain
   increasing or decreasing since injury?

3. Describe associated pain, vomiting,
   diarrhea, bloody stools, etc.

4. Other injuries, pain or ill feelings?

5. Description of health prior to injury

6. Currently taking any medications?

7. Significant history of other medical
   problems?

Objective Assessment

1. Observe:

   Client's general level of discomfort

   Alertness

   Posturing while sitting and walking

   Splinting and guarding abdomen

   Skin for wound or bruising

2. Abdominal palpation and auscultation
   should not be performed in triage

SUBJECTIVE AND OBJECTIVE DATA— GASTROINTESTINAL/ABDOMINAL TRAUMA

Signs/Symptoms

Penetrating abdominal injury

-or-

Blunt abdominal trauma within past 24 hours
Client appears ill or having significant discomfort

--YES→   CATEGORY I

Blunt abdominal trauma
No acute distress, but complains of minor discomfort
Injury within 24 hours

--YES→   CATEGORY II

Minor abdominal trauma
Client came to the emergency department just to be evaluated

--YES→   CATEGORY III

Category

ABDOMINAL TRAUMA
GASTROINTESTINAL/ABDOMINAL

8

Category I	Category II	Category III	Category IV
Abdominal pain—acute onset with vomiting, dehydration or diarrhea	Abdominal pain with rectal bleeding	Abdominal pain with vomiting and/or diarrhea client not appearing ill	Vomiting and diarrhea no signs of dehydration
Severe intermittent abdominal pain with bloody rectal mucous with or without vomiting	Client with possible appendix	Abdominal pain client with active sexual history	Constipation
	Abdominal pain, vomiting and/or diarrhea Minimal dehydration		Not eating
Severe abdominal pain with hematemesis	Rectal bleeding also having abdominal pain client appears pale	Adult with small amount rectal bleeding, fever, constipation or diarrhea	Cramps, menstrual related
Rectal bleeding or prolapse	Child under age one year rectal bleeding, fever, constipation or diarrhea		Pain upon urination Urinary frequency
Large amount bloody or tarry stool		Difficulty swallowing no swollen glands or respiratory difficulty	Rectal pain or itching
Difficulty swallowing client with respiratory distress	Difficulty swallowing, with drooling Swollen glands or tonsils		Difficulty swallowing
Navel swelling, sudden onset associated severe abdominal pain	Difficulty swallowing possible foreign body (no respiratory distress)	Minor abdominal trauma client came to emergency department just to be evaluated	Sore throat, sinus congestion
Penetrating abdominal injury	Blunt abdominal trauma no acute distress, but complains of minor discomfort Injury within past 24 hours		Chronic navel discharge, client not appearing ill
Blunt abdominal trauma within past 24 hours client appears ill or having significant discomfort			

OVERVIEW
GASTROINTESTINAL/ABDOMINAL

MAJOR SYSTEM: GENITOURINARY

Subjective and Objective Data

	Flow Sheets
Genitourinary Medical	
Female Genitourinary	Menstrual Problems
	Pregnancy
	Testicular or Penis Problems
	Inability to Urinate
	Urethral or Vaginal Discharge
	Urinary Frequency or Hematuria
Genitourinary Trauma	Genitalia Trauma
	Sexual Abuse

9

GENITOURINARY

Subjective Assessment

1. Onset of symptoms—location and description of problem.

2. Discomfort, characteristics—pain (sharp, dull, aching), cramping, urgency, burning, frequency?

3. Duration of problem—constant, intermittent?

4. Time of last voiding and symptoms associated with that voiding? Relationship of voiding with severe symptoms?

5. Characteristics of urine—blood or coke colored; clear; cloudy; concentrated?

6. Associated symptoms—costo-vertebral angle (CVA) tenderness, urethral discharge; vaginal discharge; chills; fever; backache; abdominal pain; vomiting (males—testicular pain; groin pain, radiation patterns)?

7. Current medications?

8. Previous history with similar problems? Describe.

9. Chronic diseases; self or family such as pyelonephritis, diabetes, sickle cell?

10. Evidence of possible abuse?

11. Female (see female genitourinary sheet).

12. Known exposure to venereal disease?

Objective Assessment

1. Observe client for generalized illness or discomfort.

2. Collect clean-catch urine specimen for analysis. Note gross characteristics.

SUBJECTIVE AND OBJECTIVE DATA—GENITOURINARY MEDICAL GENITOURINARY

Subjective Assessment

1. Dates and characteristics of last menstrual period.

2. Birth control measures?

3. Describe in detail:
   Pain—onset, duration, location, factors precipitating.
   Discharge—onset, amount, color, odor, associated symptoms.
   Bleeding—duration, amount (number of pads or tampons used), clots.
   Itching—location, associated rash.

4. What has client done to resolve problem?

5. Known exposure to venereal disease?

6. History of pregnancy, miscarriage, abortion?

Objective Assessment

1. If possibility of pregnancy, collect clean-catch urine for analysis and pregnancy testing.

9

SUBJECTIVE AND OBJECTIVE DATA—FEMALE GENITOURINARY GENITOURINARY

Signs/Symptoms

				Category
Vaginal hemorrhage	-or-	Vaginal bleeding, possible miscarriage Client cramping	--YES→	CATEGORY I
Vaginal bleeding Miscarriage already occurred at home			--YES→	CATEGORY II
R/O pregnancy Client having vaginal bleeding and pain			--YES→	CATEGORY III
Cramps	-or-	Client has missed period Requests evaluation for pregnancy	--YES→	CATEGORY IV

MENSTRUAL PROBLEMS
GENITOURINARY

Signs/Symptoms		X-Ray/Lab		Category
Active labor	-or-		--YES→	CATEGORY I
Vaginal bleeding, probable miscarriage				
Client with severe abdominal pain Questionable ectopic pregnancy	-or-		--YES→	CATEGORY II
Vaginal bleeding Miscarriage already occurred at home				
Client with moderate abdominal pain or cramping Questionable pregnancy		Urinalysis with pregnancy screen	--YES→	CATEGORY III
Request for pregnancy evaluation		Urinalysis with pregnancy screen	--YES→	CATEGORY IV

**PREGNANCY
GENITOURINARY**

9

Signs/Symptoms

				Category
Severe testicular pain or swelling or discoloration	-or-	Trauma to penis Client very uncomfortable	--YES→	CATEGORY I
Gross swelling of penis, more than 12 hours since last voiding Client uncomfortable	-or-	Inguinal bulge—questionable hernia Sudden onset Client in severe pain	--YES→	CATEGORY II
Swelling of penis Client able to void Minimal discomfort	-or-	Penis discharge Client uncomfortable		
		Inguinal bulge— questionable hernia Client uncomfortable	--YES→	CATEGORY III
Nonpainful swelling testicular	-or-	Penis discharge Client not uncomfortable		
		Inguinal bulge— questionable hernia— not new Client requests evaluation	--YES→	CATEGORY IV

TESTICULAR OR PENIS PROBLEM
GENITOURINARY

Signs/Symptoms

Signs/Symptoms		Category
Inability to urinate for more than 24 hours	--YES→	CATEGORY I
Inability to urinate for more than 12 hours / Client experiencing discomfort	-or-	
Possible urethral foreign body	--YES→	CATEGORY II
Inability to urinate for more than 8 hours / Client experiencing discomfort	--YES→	CATEGORY III
Child with inability to urinate for less than 8 hours	--YES→	CATEGORY IV

9

INABILITY TO URINATE
GENITOURINARY

Signs/Symptoms	X-Ray/Lab	Category
Vaginal discharge Questionable foreign body Client uncomfortable		--YES→ CATEGORY II
Urethral or vaginal discharge Client less than 10 years old No distress noted	clean-catch urinalysis	--YES→ CATEGORY III
Vaginal discharge Client older than 10 years old No distress noted -or- Itching, irritation or rash of genito- urinary area	clean-catch urinalysis	--YES→ CATEGORY IV

9

URETHRAL OR VAGINAL DISCHARGE
GENITOURINARY

Signs/Symptoms	X-Ray/Lab		Category
Hematuria or frequency Possible urinary tract infection Client uncomfortable	Clean-catch urinalysis (Save urine for culture)	--YES→	CATEGORY III
Hematuria or frequency Possible urinary tract infection No client discomfort	Clean-catch urinalysis (Save urine for culture)	--YES→	CATEGORY IV

URINARY FREQUENCY OR HEMATURIA
GENITOURINARY

9

Subjective Assessment

1. Describe injury in detail. Time since injury?

2. Associated symptoms since injury—pain (note characteristics of onset, duration, location, intensity); bleeding (characteristics of, amount, cramping); abdominal pain (note intensity, duration, characteristics of, associated vomiting or diarrhea).

3. Injury characteristics of genitalia area—lacerations, hematoma, foreign body, discoloration, bruising.

4. Is client feeling better or worse since injury?

5. Has client voided since injury? Note characteristics of urine and associated voiding problems.

6. History of possible foreign body?

7. History of similar trauma in past? Associated injury?

8. History of chronic diseases such as diabetes, urinary tract, bleeding disorders?

9. Possible sexual abuse?

Objective Assessment

1. Observe general appearance and distress of client.

2. Characteristics of hypovolemia?

3. Note characteristics of abdominal trauma such as rigidity, distension of ecchymosis.

SUBJECTIVE AND OBJECTIVE DATA—GENITOURINARY TRAUMA GENITOURINARY

206

9

Abuse as a separate area is not included in the protocols. Clients who suffer abuse will present symptoms and complaints associated with various body systems and will be triaged according to those symptoms and complaints. In the course of professional assessment the triage nurse needs to be alert to the possibility of abuse and act according to the abuse policies at the specific institution.

9

ABUSE STATEMENT
GENITOURINARY

Signs/Symptoms

Signs/Symptoms		Category
Serious injury with gross urethral or vaginal bleeding	--YES→	CATEGORY I
Trauma to labia or vaginal area with swelling, hematoma or laceration Client uncomfortable -or- Foreign body—stuck Client uncomfortable	--YES→	CATEGORY II
Minor vaginal or labia trauma No bleeding Minimal discomfort	--YES→	CATEGORY III
Foreign body—stuck Minimal discomfort	--YES→	CATEGORY IV

GENITALIA TRAUMA
GENITOURINARY

9

Signs/Symptoms		Category
Sexual abuse under 2 hours	--YES→	CATEGORY I
Possible sexual abuse, over 2 hours, less than 12 hours	--YES→	CATEGORY II
Possible sexual abuse, more than 12 hours, less than 72 hours	--YES→	CATEGORY III
Possible sexual abuse, over 72 hours	--YES→	CATEGORY IV

**SEXUAL ABUSE
GENITOURINARY**

9

9

Category I	Category II	Category III	Category IV
Severe testicular pain or swelling or discoloration	Gross swelling of penis; more than 12 hours since last voiding Client uncomfortable	Swelling of penis; unable to void; minimal discomfort	Nonpainful testicular swelling
Trauma to penis Client very uncomfortable		Penis discharge Client uncomfortable	Penis discharge Client not uncomfortable
Serious injury with gross urethral or vaginal bleeding	Inguinal bulge—questionable hernia, sudden onset Client in severe pain	Inguinal bulge—questionable hernia Client uncomfortable	Inguinal bulge—questionable hernia—not new Client requests evaluation
Inability to urinate for more than 24 hours	Trauma to labia or vaginal area with swelling, hematoma or laceration	Minor vaginal or labia trauma; no bleeding; minimal discomfort	
Sexual abuse under 2 hours	Client uncomfortable	Urethral or vaginal discharge; client less than 10 years old; no distress noted	Foreign body—stuck Minimal discomfort
Active labor	Foreign body—stuck Client uncomfortable		
Vaginal bleeding, probable miscarriage	Vaginal discharge—questionable foreign body Client uncomfortable	Inability to urinate for more than 8 hours; Client experiencing discomfort	Vaginal discharge Client older than 10 years old No distress noted
Vaginal hemorrhage			

**OVERVIEW
GENITOURINARY**

Category I	Category II	Category III	Category IV
	Inability to urinate for more than 12 hours Client experiencing discomfort	Possible sexual abuse, more than 12 hours, less than 72 hours	Itching, irritation or rash of genito-urinary area
	Possible urethral foreign body	Client with moderate abdominal pain or cramping Questionable pregnancy	Child with inability to urinate for less than 8 hours
	Possible sexual abuse, over 2 hours, less than 12 hours	R/O pregnancy, client having vaginal bleeding and pain	Possible sexual abuse, over 72 hours
	Client with severe abdominal pain, questionable ectopic pregnancy	Hematuria or frequency Possible urinary tract infection	Request for pregnancy evaluation
	Vaginal bleeding, miscarriage already occurred at home	Client uncomfortable	Cramps
			Client has missed period Request evaluation for pregnancy
			Hematuria or frequency Possible urinary tract infection No client discomfort

9

OVERVIEW (Continued)
GENITOURINARY

MAJOR SYSTEM: **HEMATOLYMPHATIC**

Subjective and Objective Data

Flow Sheets

Hematolymphatic

Hemophiliac

Sickle Cell

Swollen Lymph Nodes

10

HEMATOLYMPHATIC

Subjective Assessment

1. Describe history of current problem; onset and course of problem since onset.

2. History of chronic diseases such as bleeding disorders, sickle cell, diabetes, hypertension, etc.

3. Current medications?

4. History of similar problems? Describe.

5. Injury related to current problem? Describe.

6. If bleeding disorder—is there a history of blood in urine, stools, bloody emesis, nosebleeds, etc?

7. If sickle cell disorder—is there abdominal pain, aching joints, difficulty breathing, etc?

8. If lymphatic disorder—are there associated symptoms such as fatigue, pain, or areas of tenderness?

Objective Assessment

1. Observe general wellness or distress of client.

2. Evidence of moist, pale skin or bruising.

3. Note client posturing indicating distress or pain.

4. Note evidence of swelling that may be associated with a lymphatic problem.

SUBJECTIVE AND OBJECTIVE DATA HEMATOLYMPHATIC

Signs/Symptoms

Hemophiliac with overt bleeding

Hemophiliac with bleeding into joints or having joint pain

    – or –

Hemophiliac with history of trauma
No obvious symptoms noted

Hemophiliac with history of minor trauma
No obvious symptoms noted

Category

--YES→ CATEGORY I

--YES→ CATEGORY II

--YES→ CATEGORY III

10

HEMOPHILIAC
HEMATOLYMPHATIC

10

Signs/Symptoms | Category

Sickle cell crisis
Client with symptoms or
ischemia or hypoxia   --YES→   CATEGORY I

History of sickle cell
Client now having pain   --YES→   CATEGORY II

History of sickle cell
Client just wants to be checked
No current symptoms   --YES→   CATEGORY IV

SICKLE CELL
HEMATOLYMPHATIC

Signs/Symptoms		Category
Client with history of swollen lymph nodes Appears ill May or may not have fever	--YES→	CATEGORY III
Client with history of swollen lymph nodes Does not appear ill	--YES→	CATEGORY IV

SWOLLEN LYMPH NODES
HEMATOLYMPHATIC

10

Category I	Category II	Category III	Category IV
Hemophiliac with overt bleeding	Hemophiliac with bleeding into joints or having joint pain	Client with history of swollen lymph nodes Appears ill May or may not have fever	Client with history of swollen lymph nodes Does not appear ill
Sickle cell crisis Client with symptoms of ischemia or hypoxia	Hemophiliac with history of trauma No obvious symptoms noted	Hemophiliac with history of minor trauma No obvious symptoms noted	History of sickle cell Client just wants to be checked No current symptoms
	History of sickle cell Client now having pain		

OVERVIEW
HEMATOLYMPHATIC

MAJOR SYSTEM: INGESTIONS

Subjective and Objective Data

Flow Sheets

Accidental Poisonings   Accidental Poisonings

                               Accidental Poisoning—Food

Substance Abuse   Drug and Alcohol Abuse

11

INGESTIONS

Subjective Assessment

1. Description of poison substance.

2. Amount injected and time since ingestion.

3. First aid performed since ingestion and results of first aid treatment.

4. Description of how client has acted since ingestion—level of consciousness, respiratory status, motor coordination and strength, G.I. disturbance (vomiting, pain, diarrhea).

5. History of current or chronic health care problems.

Objective Assessment

1. Observe:

Neuro—level of consciousness, alertness anxiety, difficulty talking, swallowing, irritability, shakiness, motor strength and coordination, agitation, tremor, blurred vision

Respiratory—respiratory rate and quality, tissue oxygenation (cyanosis), breath odor

Cardiovascular—hypo- or hypertension, pulse quality

Integumentary—hue of skin, presence of rashes

2. Save urine and all emesis for toxicological analysis.

SUBJECTIVE AND OBJECTIVE DATA—ACCIDENTIAL POISONINGS INGESTIONS

Signs/Symptoms		Category
Known poison ingestion Client appearing ill May or may not have had first aid treatment	-or-	--YES→ CATEGORY I
Known poison ingestion; unknown quantity Client not ill appearing Over one hour since ingestion	-or-	--YES→ CATEGORY II
Known poison ingestion; small amount Ipecac given prior to emergency department Client has vomited, or appropriate diluent given No significant clinical signs	-or-	--YES→ CATEGORY III
History of ingestion over 12 hours ago Client not ill appearing No illness since reported ingestion Requesting evaluation	-or-	--YES→ CATEGORY IV

Category I details: Known poison ingestion / Significant quantity / No first aid treatment given

Category II details: Known poison ingestion / Significant quantity / Ipecac given prior to emergency department / Client has vomited, or appropriate diluent given / No ill appearance

Category III details: Unknown ingestion / Client not showing any adverse clinical signs at present

Category IV details: History of ingestion which is known to be nonpoisonous substance

11

ACCIDENTAL POISONINGS
INGESTIONS

Signs/Symptoms		Category
Respiratory difficulty Dysphagia, weakness, descending paralysis	--YES→	CATEGORY I
Severe nausea, vomiting, diarrhea, dehydration No respiratory involvement Client in distress	--YES→	CATEGORY II
Moderate nausea, vomiting, diarrhea, abdominal cramps, mild fever Client feels ills	--YES→	CATEGORY III
Mild nausea, abdominal cramps Client complains of not feeling well	--YES→	CATEGORY IV

ACCIDENTAL POISONING—FOOD INGESTIONS

Subjective Assessment

1. Type of substance ingestion?

2. Amount of ingestion and time since ingestion?

3. Describe course of ill feelings since ingestion.

4. Previous history of similar substance abuse and course of problem at that time?

5. History of chronic or other medical problems?

6. History of prescribed medications currently being taken?

7. If alcohol ingestion—describe drinking patterns and duration of this ingestion episode.

8. History of abdominal cramps, diarrhea, vomiting, seizure or tremors?

Objective Assessment

1. General appearance:

   Level of consciousness

   Ill state

   Amount of anxiety, irritability

   Shakiness

   Hallucinations (auditory, visual)

2. Respiratory evaluation—rate, depth and quality of respiration.

3. Cardiovascular assessment—hypo- or hypertension pulse rate and quality.

4. Is client in danger to himself or others?

SUBJECTIVE AND OBJECTIVE DATA—SUBSTANCE ABUSE INGESTIONS

11

223

Signs/Symptoms

Signs/Symptoms			Category
History of large dosage Chronic abuser; Several hours since last dose; Major withdrawal symptoms; Cardiovascular respiratory changes; hallucinating; history of seizures; feeling ill	-or-	History of large dosage with respiratory depression. Decreased level of consciousness, cardiovascular changes	--YES→ CATEGORY I
	-or-	History of ingestion; Significant behavioral changes (paranoia, severe agitation); Presents danger to self or others	
History of substance abuse; Minor withdrawal symptoms (tremors, agitation); Last dose several hours ago; Client feeling ill			--YES→ CATEGORY II
History of ingestion; Showing signs of mild intoxication or drug effect; No danger to self or others; Complains of not feeling well			--YES→ CATEGORY III

DRUG AND ALCOHOL ABUSE INGESTIONS

Category I	Category II	Category III	Category IV
History of large dosage of drug or alcohol Chronic abuser Several hours since last dose Major withdrawal symptoms	History of substance abuse Minor withdrawal symptoms (tremors, agitation) Last dose several hours ago Feeling ill	History of ingestion (alcohol/drugs) Showing signs of mild intoxication or drug effect No danger to self or others Complains of not feeling well	History of poison ingestion over 12 hours ago Client not ill appearing No illness since reported ingestion Requesting evaluation
Respiratory changes; hallucinating; history of seizures; feeling ill	Known poison ingestion: unknown quantity Client not ill appearing Over one hour since ingestion	Known poison ingestion— small amount Ipecac given prior to emergency department Client has vomited, or appropriate diluent given No significant clinical signs	History of ingestion of substance known to be nonpoisonous
History of large dosage (drug/alcohol) with respiratory depression, decreased level of consciousness; cardiovascular changes			Possible food poisoning Mild nausea, abdominal cramps Client complains of not feeling well
History of ingestion (drug/alcohol) Significant behavioral changes (Paranoia, severe agitation) Presents danger to self or others	Known poison ingestion Significant quantity Ipecac given prior to emergency department Client has vomited, or appropriate diluent given No ill appearance	Unknown ingestion of poison Client not showing any adverse clinical signs at present	

11

OVERVIEW INGESTIONS

Category I	Category II	Category III	Category IV
Known poison ingestion Client appears ill May or may not have had first aid treatment	Possible food poisoning Severe nausea, vomiting, diarrhea, dehydration No respiratory involvement Client in distress	Possible food poisoning Moderate nausea, vomiting, diarrhea, abdominal cramps, mild fever Client feels ill	
Known poison ingestion Significant quantity No first aid given			
Possible food poisoning Resiratory difficulty, dysphagia, weakness, descending paralysis			

OVERVIEW (Continued)
INGESTIONS

MAJOR SYSTEM: INTEGUMENTARY

Subjective and Objective Data

Flow Sheets

Integumentary: Bites

Human or Animal Bites

Snake, Spider, Scorpion, or
Aquatic Animal Bites

Insect Bites

Integumentary: Cold Injury

Cold Injury

Integumentary: Rash

Rash

Communicable Diseases

Integumentary: Thermal Injury

Burns

Electrical Injury

Integumentary: Trauma

Lacerations, Abrasions, Contusions

Puncture Wounds, Foreign Body

Wound Infection

12

INTEGUMENTARY

Subjective Assessment

1. Specific history related to bite attack, i.e., what, when, client's reaction within 5 minutes of bite, and in general since bite?

2. Allergic history to bites, if relevant?

3. If animal—dog, cat, rodent, etc.—description of animal, i.e., wellness; was bite agitated by client, i.e., teasing; is animal domestic—note owner identification; has animal had "shots?"

4. Spider bites—description of spider (brown recluse, black widow).

5. Snake bites—description of snake—head shape, triangular vs. oblong. History fever, nausea, vomiting generalized illness prior to or since bite (describe).

6. Human bite—description of characteristics that led to bite; description of general health of person doing the biting.

Objective Assessment

1. General observation of client.

   Allergic reaction—localized edema redness, respiratory difficulty, coughing.

   Injured area evaluation—
   severe: avulsed area
   moderate injury: multiple area involvement without avulsion: puncture wound.

   Snake bites—differentiate puncture wounds from scratch wounds, localized reaction.

   Spider bites—note localized reaction; evidence of tissue necrosis.

   Note associated generalized signs including fever, abdominal cramping, nausea, vomiting.

SUBJECTIVE AND OBJECTIVE DATA—INTEGUMENTARY: BITES
INTEGUMENTARY

Signs/Symptoms

			Category
Bite involving multiple tear lacerations or severe injury	-or-	--YES→	CATEGORY I
	Tear laceration of face: major		
Tear lacerations of face: minor		--YES→	CATEGORY II
Minor bites involving puncture wounds or break in skin		--YES→	CATEGORY III
Bites causing scratches		--YES→	CATEGORY IV

HUMAN OR ANIMAL BITES INTEGUMENTARY

12

Signs/Symptoms

Signs/Symptoms		Category
Client having much pain and appears ill	--YES→	CATEGORY I
History of spider bite, scorpion, aquatic. No current distress. Reassess client × 3 at level II, if still OK recategorize to level IV -or- History of snake bite obvious wound noted	--YES→	CATEGORY II
History of bite: client in no distress	--YES→	CATEGORY III

SNAKE/SPIDER/SCORPION/AQUATIC ANIMAL BITES
INTEGUMENTARY

Signs/Symptoms		Category
Systemic allergic response client having respiratory difficulty	-or-	--YES→ CATEGORY I
History of tick bite: client now with fever and rash		
Systemic allergic response (hives or itching), no respiratory involvement. No client distress	-or-	--YES→ CATEGORY II
Multiple bee, ant, or other insect bites		
Localized insect bites client appears well—may have local discomfort		--YES→ CATEGORY III

INSECT BITES
INTEGUMENTARY

12

Subjective Assessment

1. Describe in detail history of exposure—length of exposure; length of time since exposure.

2. Describe first aid applied.

3. Determine history of chronic diseases or circulatory problems.

4. Describe client's current symptoms—numbness vs. stinging pain.

5. Status of current tetanus immunization.

Objective Assessment

1. Observe general characteristics of injured area—color (blanched, red, bluish gray); extent of color deviation.

2. Palpate injured area to assess numbness, pain, sensation.

SUBJECTIVE AND OBJECTIVE DATA—INTEGUMENTARY: COLD INJURY INTEGUMENTARY

Signs/Symptoms		Category
Major cold injury, client has reduced core temperature	--YES→	CATEGORY I
Localized cold injury with blanching, cyanosis, or pain	--YES→	CATEGORY II
Cold injury, no discoloration, only minimal pain	--YES→	CATEGORY III

COLD INJURY
INTEGUMENTARY

12

Subjective Assessment

1. Describe in detail where the rash started and the pattern progression of the rash.

2. Exposure to communicable diseases.

3. Exposure to tick bite (time duration since bite).

4. Generalized symptoms associated?
   fever, malaise, anorexia
   headache
   abdominal pains, nausea, vomiting, diarrhea
   photophobia, conjunctivitis
   muscular aches, joint pain
   previous sore throat
   other illnesses

5. Immunizations—measles?

6. Possible allergic history—drugs, foods, household, plants, pets, etc.

7. Client history of chronic diseases.

Objective Assessment

1. Observe characteristics of rash:

   What does it look like?

   Pattern on body (describe characteristics.)

2. Observe general state of client fever.
   Conjunctivitis?

SUBJECTIVE AND OBJECTIVE DATA—INTEGUMENTARY: RASH INTEGUMENTARY

Signs/Symptoms			Category
Client with fever and petechial rash	-or-	Client with systemic rash: appears very ill --YES→	CATEGORY I
Rash—history of exposure to communicable disease	-or-	Rash (with or without blisters) client very uncomfortable and appears ill --YES→	CATEGORY II
Rash with blisters— minor discomfort reported		--YES→	CATEGORY III
Localized rash—client not appearing ill		--YES→	CATEGORY IV

**RASH
INTEGUMENTARY**

Signs/Symptoms

	Category

Communicable disease—measles, mumps, chicken pox (want to remove client from waiting room as quickly as possible)   --YES→   CATEGORY II

COMMUNICABLE DISEASE
INTEGUMENTARY

Subjective Asssessment

1. Describe in detail how burn occurred.

2. What first aid techniques have been applied?

3. Determine type of burn—flame, scald, grease, electrical, sun, tar, etc.?

4. Determine history of chronic diseases.

5. Current medications taken by client?

6. Current tetanus immunizations.

7. If flame burn, determine possibility of inhalation injury.

Objective Assessment

1. Identify amount and type of burn: Blisters and open areas versus nonblistering burn. Involvement of face, hands, feet, genitalia, neck

2. Observe burn location characteristics (abuse)?

3. Respiratory assessment to determine possibility of inhalation injury:

   Burnt nasal hairs

   Smokey color in pharynx

   Dyspnea, hoarseness

   Smokey smelling breath

12

SUBJECTIVE AND OBJECTIVE DATA—INTEGUMENTARY: THERMAL INJURY INTEGUMENTARY

12

Signs/Symptoms			Category
Major burn or full thickness burn of face, neck, hands, feet, or groin	-or-	Flame burn: possibility of inhalation injury	--YES→ CATEGORY I
Split and/or full thickness burns over less than 5% body surface area—client uncomfortable			--YES→ CATEGORY II
Split thickness burns over trunk or over more than 10% body surface area—client uncomfortable			--YES→ CATEGORY III
Split thickness burns over less than 10% body surface area—minor discomfort			--YES→ CATEGORY IV

BURNS
INTEGUMENTARY

Signs/Symptoms

			Category
Electrical and flame burn causing severe injury		--YES→	CATEGORY I
	-or-		
Flash electrical arc burn causing severe shock			
History of electrical shock burn, only surface damage noted		--YES→	CATEGORY II

ELECTRICAL INJURY
INTEGUMENTARY

12

Subjective Assessment

1. Description of exactly what happened, where, when, and how? Time duration since injury. Possible missile injury? If so, character, direction and force of missile?

2. Tetanus immunization history?

3. First aid applied?

4. History of possible foreign body in wound?

5. History of bleeding or clotting difficulties?

6. Overall wellness of client?

7. History of multiple bruises, or unrelated injuries (abuse)?

Objective Assessment

1. Observe wound area for:
   Extent of injury
   Cleanliness vs. contamination
   Active bleeding
   Infection

2. Observe overall state of client, i.e., multiple bruises or bruises at different healing states.

3. Observe response as client is requested to move injured area through active range of motion (tendon/muscle evaluation).

4. Observe and palpate area distal to injury to evaluate neural intactness, bone injury, foreign body, arterial and venous flow.

SUBJECTIVE AND OBJECTIVE DATA—INTEGUMENTARY TRAUMA INTEGUMENTARY

Signs/Symptoms | Category

Signs/Symptoms			Category
Active bleeding, unable to control bleeding	-or-	Laceration with severe nerve tendon or vascular injury	--YES→ CATEGORY I
Laceration bleeding requiring pressure dressing	-or-	Tendon injury or nerve injury or significant crush injury	--YES→ CATEGORY II
Laceration—uncomplicated no bleeding—will require sutures	-or-	Minor crush injury—no current distress noted	--YES→ CATEGORY III
Abrasions, contusions, split thickness lacerations may not require suturing			--YES→ CATEGORY IV

12

LACERATIONS/ABRASIONS/CONTUSIONS INTEGUMENTARY

12

PUNCTURE WOUNDS/FOREIGN BODY INTEGUMENTARY

Signs/Symptoms	X-Ray/Lab		Category
Foreign body due to missile: object still in place—client having distress		--YES→	CATEGORY I
Foreign body—object in place, client uncomfortable—but no distress noted	X-ray for foreign body location	--YES→	CATEGORY II
Puncture wound—questionable foreign body in place	X-ray for foreign body	--YES→	CATEGORY III
Minor small puncture wound		--YES→	CATEGORY IV

Signs/Symptoms		Category
Infected wound, client ill appearing		
-or-		
Cellulitis of face or periorbital area	--YES→	CATEGORY I
Cellulitis client appears ill and has over 103° temperature	--YES→	CATEGORY II
Localized wound infection— client appears well. Example, impetigo or pus in wound		
-or-		
Localized cellulitis	--YES→	CATEGORY III
Suture removal	--YES→	CATEGORY IV

**WOUND INFECTION
INTEGUMENTARY**

12

Category I	Category II	Category III	Category IV
Bite—multilacerations or severe injury	Bite—minor tear laceration of face	Minor bites involving puncture wound or break in skin	Bite causing scratches
Tear laceration of face	History of snake or spider bite—no distress, but wound obvious	Minor uncomplicated lacerations	Localized insect bites
Snake bite—client ill, having much pain		Minor crush injury	Abrasions, contusions
Insect bite—systemic allergic response—respiratory difficulty	Insect bite—systemic minor allergic response		Minor puncture wound
	Multiple bee or insect bites	Puncture wound? Foreign body	Localized wound infection; client appears well
History of tick bite—client now ill, with rash and fever	Laceration requiring pressure to contain bleeding	Rash with blisters; minor discomfort reported.	Localized cellulitis
Trauma—active bleeding unable to control	Significant crush injury, minor discomfort	Cold injury—no discoloration; only minimal pain	Suture removal
Laceration with severe nerve tendon or vascular injury	Foreign body—object still in place; no client distress noted	Split thickness burns over trunk or over more than 10% body surface area; minor discomfort	Client with localized rash
Puncture wound and foreign body due to missile injury; client in distress	Cellulitis—client appearing ill		Split thickness burn over less than 10% body surface area—minor discomfort

**OVERVIEW
INTEGUMENTARY**

Category I	Category II	Category III	Category IV
Infected wound—client appears ill	Rash—history of exposure to communicable disease		
Client with cellulitis of face or priorbital area	Known communicable disease		
Client with rash—appears very ill and toxic	Rash—client appears ill		
Client with fever and petechial rash	Localized cold injury with blanching, cyanosis or pain		
Major cold injury—client with reduced core temp.	Split and/or full thickness burns over less than 5%		
Major burn or full thickness burn of face, neck, hands, feet, groin	body surface area—client uncomfortable		
Flame burn—possible inhalation injury	History of electrical injury, only minor burn noted		
Electrical burns—significant shock/injury			

OVERVIEW (Continued)
INTEGUMENTARY

12

MAJOR SYSTEM: MOUTH AND THROAT

Subjective and Objective Data

Mouth and Throat

Flow Sheets

Mouth Sores

Mouth Trauma

Sore Throat, Hoarseness, Swollen
Glands, Laryngitis

T and A Bleeder

13

MOUTH AND THROAT

Subjective Assessment

1. Describe details of current complaint.
2. Duration of problem.
3. Trauma involved. Describe (mouth-throat).
4. Other systemic symptoms:
   Headaches
   Dizziness
   Muscular ache
   Weakness
   Fever
   Allergy, hay fever, nasal problems
   Nausea/vomiting
5. Others with similar symptoms at home?
6. Current medications.
7. Fluid and food intake.
8. Recent surgery involving mouth or throat (T&A, tooth extraction, etc.).

Objective Assessment

1. Observe client for general distress, difficulty swallowing, or drooling.
2. Observe and note characteristics (swelling, lesions, pustules, color, punctures) of lips; buccal mucosa; gingiva; tongue; tonsillar pillar; tonsils; posterior pharynx.
3. Palpate cervical lymph nodes to evaluate presence and characteristics.
4. Evaluate client's ability to talk (hoarseness?).
5. Evaluate presence of dehydration.
6. Evaluate adequacy of client's respiratory function (stridor, retractions, nasal flaring).

**SUBJECTIVE AND OBJECTIVE DATA
MOUTH AND THROAT**

248

13

Child—appears ill and dehydrated
Multiple mouth sores
Herpes gingivastomatitis

-or-

Tonsil pustules
Client very uncomfortable
Difficulty swallowing
May be drooling

--YES→   CATEGORY II

Child—herpes gingivastomatitis
history
No fluids for 12 hours
Fever

-or-

Multiple mouth or tonsil
pustules
Client uncomfortable

--YES→   CATEGORY III

Multiple minor mouth sores

-or-

Child with "cottage cheese"
spots in mouth

--YES→   CATEGORY IV

MOUTH SORES
MOUTH AND THROAT

13

Signs/Symptoms

		Category
Amputated tongue tip or large section of cheek		
-or-		
Hoarseness with history of trauma to larynx	--YES→	CATEGORY I
Puncture wound, soft palate	--YES→	CATEGORY II
Partial tongue laceration or cheek bite		
-or-		
Puncture wound, hard palate	--YES→	CATEGORY III

MOUTH TRAUMA
MOUTH AND THROAT

Signs/Symptoms				Category
Sore throat with drooling Inspirator/expiratory stridor, elevated temperature and ill appearing	-or-	Hoarse cry in baby under 3 months of age Elevated temperature	-or-	Sudden onset of hoarseness Difficulty swallowing and/or breathing	--YES→	CATEGORY I
Sore throat with fever over 101°	-or-	Laryngitis with fever over 101°	-or-	Swollen glands with fever over 101°	--YES→	CATEGORY III
Sore throat with fever under 101°	-or-	Laryngitis with fever under 101°	-or-	Swollen glands with fever under 101°	--YES→	CATEGORY IV

SORE THROAT/HOARSENESS/SWOLLEN GLANDS/LARYNGITIS MOUTH AND THROAT

13

Signs/Symptoms	X-Ray/Lab		Category
Active bleeding Client appears pale		--YES→	CATEGORY I
T&A bleeder by history No active bleeding Client appears pale	Hematocrit Hemoglobin	--YES→	CATEGORY II

T&A BLEEDER
MOUTH AND THROAT

Category I	Category II	Category III	Category IV
Trauma:			
Amputated tongue tip or large section of cheek	Puncture wound of soft palate	Partial tongue laceration or cheek bite	
Hoarseness with history of trauma to larynx		Puncture wound hard palate	
Medical:	Child:	Child:	
T&A bleeder Active bleeding Client appears pale	Herpes gingivastomatitis Child ill and dehydrated	Herpes gingivastomatitis history No fluids for 12 hours	Multiple minor mouth sores
Sore throat with drooling and stridor Client ill appearing	Tonsil pustules Difficulty swallowing Client very uncomfortable	Multiple mouth or tonsil pustules Client uncomfortable	Child with cottage cheese spots in mouth
Hoarse cry in baby under 3 months old Elevated temperature	T&A bleeder by history No active bleeding Client appears pale	Sore throat with fever over 101°	Sore throat with fever under 101°
Sudden onset of hoarseness Difficulty breathing and swallowing		Laryngitis with fever over 101°	Laryngitis with fever under 101°
		Swollen glands with fever over 101°	Swollen glands with fever under 101°

13

OVERVIEW
MOUTH AND THROAT

MAJOR SYSTEM: MUSCULOSKELETAL

Subjective and Objective Data

Flow Sheets

Musculoskeletal Medical

Extremity Pain
Joint Pain
Muscle Ache or Muscle Problem

Musculoskeletal Trauma

Amputation
Cast Problems
Cervical or Back Injury
Crush Injury
Dislocations
Fractures
Hemophiliac with Musculoskeletal Injury
Physical Abuse

Criteria for X-Ray Evaluation

MUSCULOSKELETAL

14

Subjective Assessment

1. Describe problem in detail.

2. Is there history of similar problem?

3. Has there been an unrelated illness or injury during the past several weeks (e.g., strep throat, rheumatic fever)?

4. Is there a history of chronic disease (e.g., sickle cell, osteomyletis, rheumatoid, arthritis, hemophilia)?

5. What other systemic problems are present (e.g., fever, chills, malaise, anorexia)?

6. What current medications are being taken?

7. History of muscle spasms?

8. History of drug ingestion?

Objective Assessment

1. Observe area of concern for contour, color (redness), and swelling.

2. Observe how client uses affected area:
   Is client using or not using affected area?
   Is there guarding of affected area?

3. Palpate affected area to evaluate:
   Range of motion
   Tenderness
   Swelling
   Joint effusion
   Heat of joint or area
   Pain or discomfort of area with movement

SUBJECTIVE AND OBJECTIVE DATA— MUSCULOSKELETAL MEDICAL MUSCULOSKELETAL

Signs/Symptoms		Category
Severe extremity pain with absence of extremity pulse or with limb discoloration	--YES→	CATEGORY II
Extremity pain Client appears ill, has history of fever or other systemic illness	--YES→	CATEGORY III
Vague extremity pain or stiffness Client does not appear ill	--YES→	CATEGORY IV

EXTREMITY PAIN MUSCULOSKELETAL

14

Signs/Symptoms

		Category
Joint pain with obvious dislocation	--YES→	CATEGORY I
Joint pain with fever over 102° (children's fever over 100°) or known hemophilia -or- Swollen "hot" joint Client appears ill May or may not have fever	--YES→	CATEGORY II
Swollen "hot"joint No fever Client appears well	--YES→	CATEGORY III
Vague complaint of joint pain Client appears in no distress	--YES→	CATEGORY IV

14

258

**JOINT PAIN
MUSCULOSKELETAL**

Signs/Symptoms		Category
Severe muscle cramps Client showing significant discomfort, may or may not have fever -or- Child: Muscle weakness Client appears ill May have fever	--YES→	CATEGORY II
Minor or vague muscle cramps not interfering with overall client comfort -or- Muscle weakness Client appears ill May have fever	--YES→	CATEGORY III
Minor or vague muscle discomforts	--YES→	CATEGORY IV

MUSCLE ACHE OR MUSCLE PROBLEM
MUSCULOSKELETAL

14

Subjective Assessment

1. Describe injury in detail. Describe mechanism of injury and direction of force.

2. Time elapse since injury? First aid treatment?

3. Ability to move or use extremity since injury. Describe.

4. History of other injuries (e.g., abdomen, head, other musculoskeletal injuries)?

5. Current medications?

6. Chronic diseases (e.g., hemophilia).

7. History of previous and similar musculoskeletal injuries?

8. History of possible physical abuse?

Objective Assessment

1. Observe trauma area—note deformity, skin break (open?), dislocation, color distal to injury, abnormal position of limb, swelling.

2. Evaluate the 5 Ps associated with the injury:
   Pain (note location and precipitating factors)
   Pulses (distal to injury, compare bilaterally)
   Paresthesia (numbness or diminished sensation)
   Paralysis (associated with injured part)
   Pallor (distal to injury, compare bilaterally)

3. Gently manipulate extremity to evaluate range of motion.

4. Palpate to determine specific area of injury.

SUBJECTIVE AND OBJECTIVE DATA—MUSCULOSKELETAL TRAUMA MUSCULOSKELETAL

The triage nurse will initiate x-ray evaluation of the following area to determine the possibilities of fractures:

Fingers   Clavicle
Hands   Feet
Wrists   Ankle
Forearm   Tibia/fibula
Elbow   Knee
Humerous   Femur
Shoulder   Skull

Criteria for determination of x-ray:

YES (order x-ray)

a. Definite deformity

b. Pain with attempt of manipulation

c. Unable to bear weight or to use extremity

d. Pain with direct palpation

e. Client requests x-ray

NO X-RAY

a. Category I client

b. Full range of motion without discomfort

c. No pain with direct palpation even though swelling may be present

d. Able to use extremity, bear weight

X-RAY CRITERIA MUSCULOSKELETAL

14

Signs/Symptoms		X-Ray/Lab		Category
Traumatic amputation Active bleeding or client with amputated part			--YES→	CATEGORY I
-or-				
Traumatic injury major portion of limb (hand, foot)				
Traumatic amputation of distal digit Amputated part not available for reattachment No bleeding		X-ray of injured limb	--YES→	CATEGORY II

14

AMPUTATION
MUSCULOSKELETAL

Signs/Symptoms		Category
Tight cast with neurovascular impairment	--YES→	CATEGORY II
Broken casts Cast needing reinforcement	--YES→	CATEGORY IV

CAST PROBLEMS
MUSCULOSKELETAL

14

Signs/Symptoms

Cervical or back pain
with history of significant
trauma

--YES→

Category

CATEGORY I

Minor back problem or trauma
related to "I pulled something"
No acute distress

--YES→

CATEGORY III

Muscle ache without
other symptoms

--YES→

CATEGORY IV

CERVICAL OR BACK INJURY
MUSCULOSKELETAL

14

Signs/Symptoms

Crush or wringer injury
Client in pain
Injury obvious

--YES→

Category

CATEGORY I

History of crush injury
Minimal injury
Client in slight discomfort

--YES→

CATEGORY II

CRUSH INJURY
MUSCULOSKELETAL

14

14

Signs/Symptoms		Category
Obvious dislocation	--YES→	CATEGORY I
History of dislocation, but no current signs See fracture protocol	--YES→	CATEGORY III

DISLOCATIONS
MUSCULOSKELETAL

Signs/Symptoms	X-Ray/Lab	Category
Open fracture break in skin over possible fracture site -or- Probable fracture femur -or- Possible fracture with circulatory or neural impairment		--YES→ CATEGORY I
Probable extremity fracture	Splint and x-ray See x-ray criteria	--YES→ CATEGORY II
Possible extremity fracture	Splint and x-ray See x-ray criteria	--YES→ CATGORY III
Bump to extremities without swelling		--YES→ CATEGORY IV

FRACTURES
MUSCULOSKELETAL

14

MUSCULOSKELETAL
HEMOPHILIAC WITH MUSCULOSKELETAL INJURY

Signs/Symptoms		Category
Client with known hemophilia, obvious musculoskeletal injury with bleeding into tissue	--YES→	CATEGORY I
Client with known hemophilia, history of musculoskeletal injury No active signs of bleeding into tissue	--YES→	CATEGORY II

REMAIN ALERT FOR POSSIBLE PHYSICAL ABUSE

Red Flags Include:

1. History of injury does not coincide with injury itself.

2. There has been a delay in seeking treatment.

3. Family member seems overly concerned or lacks concern about client's injury.

4. Multiple bruises in association with or separate from injury.

Specifics for Children:

1. Note interaction of child and parent.

2. Observe behavior of child (blank stare, doesn't cry when approached, lies very still).

3. Lack of development of child.

4. Evidence of previous injuries.

5. Injury cannot be explained by parents.

* Because of type of problem—Category II for all possible abuse clients

PHYSICAL ABUSE
MUSCULOSKELETAL

14

Category I	Category II	Category III	Category IV
Open fracture	Probable extremity fracture	Muscle spasms	Localized back pain, not trauma related
Probable femur fracture with difference in thigh diameter	Multiple joint pain with fever	Minor back problems, trauma related, i.e., "pulled something"	Bump to extremities without swelling
Any possible fracture with circulatory or neural impairment	Hip pain with fever	Possible extremity fracture	Muscle ache without other symptoms
	Tight cast with neurological or vascular impairment	Swollen "hot" joint	
Crush injury—significant	Possibly abused client	Tight cast with edema	
Obvious dislocation	History hemophilia	Muscle ache with fever	
Any cervical or back pain with history of significant trauma	No noted injury		
	Extremity pain, client appears ill		
Traumatic amputations	Severe muscle cramps		
Hemophiliac with obvious injury			
Severe extremity pain with circulatory compromise			

OVERVIEW
MUSCULOSKELETAL

MAJOR SYSTEM: NEUROLOGICAL

Subjective and Objective Data	Flow Sheets
Neurological Medical	Confusion
	Fainting
	Headache
	Irritable Child
	Motor Weakness (Possible CVA)
	Seizure, Seizure Disorder
	Shunt Dysfunction
Neurological Trauma	Hit Head, Head Trauma, Neck Injury
	Low Back Injury, Low Back Pain

NEUROLOGICAL

15

271

Subjective Assessment

1. History of possible injury? Describe in detail (move to trauma questions).

2. History of similar problem (i.e., seizure)? Precipitating factors.

3. If seizure, describe exactly what happened.

4. History of illness? Self—family (describe).

5. History of possible ingestion?

6. History of chronic diseases (i.e., seizure disorder, diabetes, shunt dysfunction).

7. History of current medications?

8. History of selected systems:
   Neuro—headaches, neck pains, weakness, paralysis, vertigo, light headedness, staggering gait
   G.I.—vomiting, nausea, diarrhea
   Integument—rash (note characteristics)

9. History of drowsiness, confusion?

10. What changes have there been in client's health state during past 6 hours, 24 hours, week?

Objective Assessment

1. Observe client's overall alertness. If client is child, note irritability, lethargy, or ill appearance.

2. Observe client's gait and gross motor functioning.

3. Observe purposeful fine motor movement.

4. Evaluate speech pattern and clarity of tone.

5. Evaluate client's orientation to person, place and thing. Is client able to follow directions?

6. Special for Children (assessment for meningeal signs):
   Fontanelle bulge
   Paradoxical irritability—child cries when held
   Kernig's sign—bend thigh at hip and attempt to extend leg at knee (increased pain—positive sign)
   Brudzinski's sign—bend neck with child supine (knees bend spontaneously—positive sign)

SUBJECTIVE AND OBJECTIVE DATA— NEUROLOGICAL MEDICAL NEUROLOGICAL

Signs/Symptoms

		Category
Sudden onset of confusion associated with altered sensorium	--YES→	CATEGORY I
Sudden onset of confusion associated with weakness, headache or other neurological signs	--YES→	CATEGORY II
Client showing confusion state, which interferes with activities of daily living No acute distress (evaluate for substance abuse)	--YES→	CATEGORY III

**CONFUSION
NEUROLOGICAL**

15

Signs/Symptoms

		Category
History of fainting Now showing altered consciousness state or other neurological symptoms	--YES→	CATEGORY I
History of fainting Hit head Now feeling ill or having severe headache	--YES→	CATEGORY II
History of fainting Still not feeling well Vague complaints No acute distress	--YES→	CATEGORY III

FAINTING
NEUROLOGICAL

Signs/Symptoms

		Category
Severe headache with disorientation or elevated blood pressure -or- History of severe headache Now showing altered sensorium	--YES→	CATEGORY I
Severe headache History of head trauma within past 2 weeks -or- Irritable child with meningeal signs -or- Sudden onset of headache unlike any client has had before with or without vomiting	--YES→	CATEGORY II
Chronic headache or similar type headache that client has had before Client not in distress	--YES→	CATEGORY III
Minor headache, not interfering with client's activities of daily living	--YES→	CATEGORY IV

HEADACHE
NEUROLOGICAL

15

Signs/Symptoms

Signs/Symptoms				Category
Does not respond to verbal stimuli (doesn't recognize mother)	-or-	Possible ingestion	-or- Dextrostix 0–45	--YES→ CATEGORY I
Irritable with fever	-or-	Dextrostix 45–90	--YES→	CATEGORY II
Irritable No other findings			--YES→	CATEGORY III

IRRITABLE CHILD
NEUROLOGICAL

Signs/Symptoms		Category
Severe motor weakness, sudden onset Client appears ill Unilateral or bilateral weakness or numbness (possible stroke)	--YES→	CATEGORY I
Recent period of significant motor weakness or numbness or tingling sensation with or without orientation Client appears weak or ill	--YES→	CATEGORY II
Vague complaints of weakness Client appears ill or unsteady	--YES→	CATEGORY III
Vague complaints of tiredness or weakness No acute distress	--YES→	CATEGORY IV

MOTOR WEAKNESS (POSSIBLE CVA)
NEUROLOGICAL

15

Signs/Symptoms

Signs/Symptoms			Category
Active seizure or postseizure state	-or-	History of seizure type activity Possibility of ingestion	--YES→ CATEGORY I
Known seizure disorder Seizure activity prior to E.D. visit. No seizure activity at present	-or-	Children with irritability and vomiting No seizure history (Dextrostix 45–90)	--YES→ CATEGORY II
Known seizure disorder No seizure activity today but "feels funny"			--YES→ CATEGORY III

SEIZURE/SEIZURE DISORDER
NEUROLOGICAL

Signs/Symptoms

Signs/Symptoms		Category
Shunt dysfunction Client appears ill History of vomiting or dehydration	--YES→	CATEGORY I
Shunt dysfunction Client is irritable but not acutely ill	--YES→	CATEGORY II

SHUNT DYSFUNCTION NEUROLOGICAL

15

Subjective Assessment

1. History of injury—describe in detail. What happened? How long ago? Distance fallen? Object struck? Loss of consciousness?

2. How did client look immediately following injury (unconscious, dazed, crying, convulsion)? Describe.

3. How was he five minutes later (vomiting, headache, O.K., no change)?

4. Nosebleed or drainage from ears?

5. Increased sleepiness?

6. Gait problems?

7. Any complaints of vision problems (droopy eyes, blurred, double vision)?

8. Vomiting? Describe style and number of times.

9. Prior neurological disorders (seizures)?

10. Current medications? Describe.

Objective Assessment

1. Identification of obvious wounds.

2. Scalp evaluation, screen for hematoma, lacerations, abrasions.

3. Observation of client in general: alertness, ability to follow directions, sleepiness, irritability

4. Respiratory evaluation (depth and pattern).

5. Can client state what happened?

6. Gait evaluation, able to walk?

7. Cranial nerve evaluation:
   II—visual acuity
   III, IV, VI—eye movements in all fields of gaze
   V—corneal reflex, clench teeth
   VII—symmetry of face, smile, raise eyebrows, puff out cheek
   VIII—hearing
   IX, X—gag reflex
   XI—shrug shoulders
   XII—tongue protusion

SUBJECTIVE AND OBJECTIVE DATA—NEUROLOGICAL TRAUMA NEUROLOGICAL

Signs/Symptoms	X-Ray/Lab		Category
Major head and/or neck injury		--YES→	CATEGORY I
History of head/neck trauma with reported unconsciousness (any time within past 2 weeks) Client now showing positive neurological signs			
Hit head with reported unconsciousness, or stunned, or vomited more than 3 times	(Physician should evaluate client prior to skull x-rays)	--YES→	CATEGORY II
Hit head, no loss of consciousness Fell significant distance or hit head very hard	Skull x-rays	--YES→	CATEGORY III
Minor head bump May have hematoma		--YES→	CATEGORY IV

HIT HEAD/HEAD TRAUMA/NECK INJURY NEUROLOGICAL

15

15

Signs/Symptoms

Signs/Symptoms		Category
Sudden onset lower back pain following bending or injury. Numbness or tingling of lower extremities. Client in great deal of pain		
-or-		
Sudden severe change in chronic low back pain situation. Client in distress	--YES→	CATEGORY I
Sudden onset lower back pain following bending or injury Vague and minor complaints of strain	--YES→	CATEGORY II
Chronic low back pain or spasm causing client minor discomfort	--YES→	CATEGORY III or IV

LOW BACK INJURY/LOW BACK PAIN
NEUROLOGICAL

Category I	Category II	Category III	Category IV
Trauma			
Major head injury	Hit head	Hit head	Minor head bump
Neck injury	Now vomiting	No loss of consciousness	
Hit head within past 2 weeks—now showing neurological signs			
Sudden onset low back pain	Sudden onset low back pain	Chronic low back pain or spasm causing minor discomfort	
Client in distress	Vague minor complaints		
Sudden change in chronic low back pain status			
Medical			
Sudden onset of confusion associated with altered sensorium	Sudden onset confusion associated with weakness or headache	Client demonstrating confusion	
		Slow onset interfering with activities of daily living	
History of fainting	History of fainting	History of fainting	
Now showing altered state of consciousness	Now feeling ill, has headache	Still not feeling well	
Severe motor weakness	Recent period of significant motor weakness with or without disorientation	Vague complaints of weakness or not feeling well	Vague complaints of tiredness or weakness
Sudden onset		Client unsteady	No acute distress
Client appears ill (possible stroke)			

OVERVIEW
NEUROLOGICAL

15

Category I	Category II	Category III	Category IV
Shunt dysfunction Client appears ill	Shunt dysfunction Client irritable but not acutely ill		
Child irritable, doesn't respond	Child irritable with fever	Child irritable No other findings	
Irritable child Possible drug ingestion	Child irritable Dextrostix 45–90		
Irritable child Dextrostix 0–45			
Active seizure state History of seizure Possible ingestion	Known seizure disorder Seizure prior to emergency department visit No seizure at present	Known seizure disorder No seizure today, but reports feeling funny	
Severe headache with high blood pressure or disorientation	Severe headache History of head trauma during past two weeks	Chronic headache or repeating type headache Client in no acute distress	Minor headache
History severe headache Now showing altered sensorium	Irritable child with meningeal signs		
	Sudden onset of headache like client has never had before		

OVERVIEW (Continued)
NEUROLOGICAL

Subjective and Objective Data

Flow Sheets

Nose and Nasal

Epistaxis

Foreign Body

Hay Fever, Allergy, Sinus

Nose Trauma

NOSE AND NASAL

16

Subjective Assessment

1. History of nose trauma?

2. If bleeding, history of similar problems in past? Frequency, duration?

3. History of high blood pressure in family?

4. Bleeding disorders—self? family?

5. Possibility of foreign body in nose (playing with small toys)?

6. Current medications?

7. If bleeding, what first aid techniques have been tried?

8. Any other systemic problems—cold, temperature, congestion?

9. History of allergies—hay fever, etc.

10. Children—history of nose picking.

Objective Assessment

1. General observation of nose. If trauma, note swelling, contour, color, lesions.

2. Bleeding?

3. Respiratory assessment—including patency of nasal passages.

4. Observe nostrils for patency.

SUBJECTIVE AND OBJECTIVE DATA
NOSE AND NASAL

Signs/Symptoms		X-Ray/Lab		Category
History of high blood pressure, or headache or not feeling well Now persistent nosebleed Denies trauma to nose	-or- Epistaxis with persistent bleeding -or- Bloody drainage from nose following trauma		--YES→	CATEGORY I
Intermittent bleeding with trauma history	-or- Intermittent bleeding with history of high blood pressure	Nasal films for clients with nasal trauma	--YES→	CATEGORY II
Periodic epistaxis with fever			--YES→	CATEGORY III
Epistaxis with nose picking			--YES→	CATEGORY IV

EPISTAXIS
NOSE AND NASAL

16

Signs/Symptoms

Category

Small foreign body in nose
that could be aspirated   --YES→   CATEGORY II

Foreign body in nose
Complains of pain   --YES→   CATEGORY III

Foreign body in nose
No discomfort   --YES→   CATEGORY IV

FOREIGN BODY
NOSE AND NASAL

16

Signs/Symptoms		Category
History of chronic lung or breathing problem Now having some congestion due to hay fever or allergy	--YES→	CATEGORY II
Allergy or hay fever causing nasal congestion	--YES→	CATEGORY III
Sinus problem	--YES→	CATEGORY IV

HAY FEVER/ALLERGY/SINUS NOSE AND NASAL

16

Signs/Symptoms	X-Ray/Lab		Category
Bloody or clear drainage from nose following head trauma		--YES→	CATEGORY I
Hit in nose Now having some nasal-respiratory difficulties Deformity noted	Nasal x-ray	--YES→	CATEGORY II
Hit in nose No respiratory difficulties Has swelling or deformity of nose	Nasal x-ray	--YES→	CATEGORY III

NOSE TRAUMA
NOSE AND NASAL

Category I	Category II	Category III	Category IV
Bloody or clear drainage from nose following head trauma	Hit in nose Now having some nasal/ respiratory difficulty	Foreign body in nose Client complains of pain	Sinus problems
History of high blood pressure, or headache or not feeling well Now persistent nosebleed Denies trauma to nose	Epistaxis with trauma History of elevated blood pressure Intermittent bleeding	Hit in nose, no respiratory difficulty	Epistaxis with nose picking
Epistaxis with persistent bleeding	History chronic lung or breathing problem Now having some congestion due to hay fever or allergy	Allergy–hay fever Causing nasal congestion	Foreign body in nose No discomfort
	Small foreign body in nose that could be aspirated	Periodic epistaxis with fever	
	Intermittent bleeding with trauma history		

OVERVIEW
NOSE AND NASAL

16

MAJOR SYSTEM: PSYCHOLOGICAL STRESS

Subjective and Objective Data   **Flow Sheets**

Psychological Stress   Psychological Stress

PSYCHOLOGICAL STRESS

Subjective Assessment

1. Reason client has come to the emergency department? Precipitating event.

2. Associated history with drugs or alcohol (see toxicology assessment).

3. Identification of major stressors including origin, number and duration.

4. Determine degree of perceived threat.

5. Describe associated feelings (i.e., chest pressure, choking, palpitations, fatigue, helplessness, vertigo, fear of losing control, etc.).

6. Previous similar episodes? Significant past medical history. Significant psychological history

7. Current medications.

Objective Assessment

1. Evaluate client's vital signs. Evaluate hyperventilation and tachycardia.

2. Observe—skin for coldness or clammy texture; facial expression for rigidity or flat affect; body position for rigidity, tremors, ataxia, or slumped posture.

3. Assess cognitive process—scattered, fragmented, illogical, irrational; memory deficit, hallucinations.

4. Assess behavioral state—confused, disoriented, agitated, combative, restless, withdrawn, having outbursts.

5. Assess tremors or seizure.

SUBJECTIVE AND OBJECTIVE DATA
PSYCHOLOGICAL STRESS

Signs/Symptoms			Category
Client known attempted suicide Psychologically unstable	-or-	--YES→	CATEGORY I
Significant subjective and/or objective data indicating that client may be dangerous to himself or others, or extremely agitated			
Client agitated or depressed Alone in waiting room Needs close observation		--YES→	CATEGORY II
Client with multiple signs and symptoms Cooperative, desires help and assessment		--YES→	CATEGORY III
Repeated use of emergency department for minor or chronic disturbances		--YES→	CATEGORY IV

PSYCHOLOGICAL STRESS

17

Category I	Category II	Category III	Category IV
Client known attempted suicide	Client agitated or depressed—alone in waiting room	Current multiple symptoms No acute distress but client desires assessment	Repeated use of emergency facility for minor or chronic disturbances
Psychologically unstable	Needs close observation		
Significant subjective and/or objective data indicating that client is extremely agitated or may be dangerous to himself or others			

OVERVIEW
PSYCHOLOGICAL STRESS

MAJOR SYSTEM: RESPIRATORY

Subjective and Objective Data

Flow Sheets

Respiratory

Breathing Difficulties, Chest Pain

Chest Trauma

Congested, Cold

Cough

Croup-Type Cough

Hemoptysis

Hyperventilation

Inhalation Injury

Possible Foreign Body Aspiration

Rib Pain

Shortness of Breath

Tracheostomy

Wheeze

RESPIRATORY

18

Subjective Assessment

1. History of previous episodes or chronic problems. History of high blood pressure.

2. Currently taking medication for respiratory problem (OTC, Rx.).

3. Characteristics of problem—cough frequency, duration of cough, dry versus productive (characteristics of sputum).

4. Dyspnea? Continuous versus activity related.

5. Possible aspiration?

6. Fatigue, listlessness—describe.

7. Allergy history—environmental, foods, drugs.

8. Chest pains—describe relationship to:
   Cough or deep breath
   Twisting of thorax
   Point tenderness to touch

9. History of chronic diseases such as respiratory, cardiovascular.

10. Smoking history—amount, kind.

11. Previous lung or heart surgery.

Objective Assessment

1. Observe overall appearance of client. Note distress, diaphoresis, ill appearance.

2. Observe:
   Inspiratory respiratory movement
   Contour and symmetry of breathing
   Nasal flaring
   Cyanosis—general versus distal, circumoral
   General breathing difficulty
   Noise with breathing, inspiratory stridor
   Drooling
   Rate and rhythm of respiration

3. Auscultation:
   Noise with respiration (throughout, unilateral, tracheal)
   Decreased breathing sounds (throughout, unilateral, tracheal)

4. Evaluate blood pressure—respiration rate, depth, quality.

SUBJECTIVE AND OBJECTIVE DATA RESPIRATORY

Signs/Symptoms | Category

Signs/Symptoms			Category
Breathing difficulty Cyanosis Periods of apnea Decreased or absence of breathing sounds Any cardiac history	-or-	Irritable, hypoxic Client appears ill May have history of chronic lung problem	--YES→ CATEGORY I
Infant: mild nasal flare See-saw breathing Child irritable			--YES→ CATEGORY II
Client complains of chest pains with breathing No cardiac history Client may have congestion or fever No acute distress noted			--YES→ CATEGORY III
Mild congestion or breathing difficulty No fever Client does not appear ill			--YES→ CATEGORY IV

BREATHING DIFFICULTIES/CHEST PAIN RESPIRATORY

18

Signs/Symptoms

Signs/Symptoms		Category
Penetrating or blunt chest trauma Client now showing signs of respiratory distress	--YES→	CATEGORY I
Blunt chest injury Client complains of rib pain No respiratory distress (see rib pain protocol)	--YES→	CATEGORY III
Minor chest trauma Bruising may be present, but no specific rib or breathing difficulties	--YES→	CATEGORY IV

18

CHEST TRAUMA
RESPIRATORY

Signs/Symptoms

Signs/Symptoms		Category
Breathing difficulties Cyanosis Periods of apnea Decreased breathing sounds Any cardiac history	-or- Irritable, hypoxic child Client appears ill	--YES→ CATEGORY I
Infant under 6 months of age: Mild nasal flaring See-saw breathing	-or- Chronic breathing problems Now has congestion and difficulty breathing	--YES→ CATEGORY II
Congested, feeling ill Fever over 101° more than 24 hours		--YES→ CATEGORY III
Congested Fever less than 101°	-or- Stuffy or runny nose	--YES→ CATEGORY IV

CONGESTED/COLD RESPIRATORY

18

Signs/Symptoms

Signs/Symptoms		Category
Continuous cough Client exhausted or in respiratory distress	-or-	
Cough causing distress Client with history of cardiac or chronic lung problem	--YES→	CATEGORY I
Cough Possibility of aspiration No immediate distress noted	--YES→	CATEGORY II
Cough Productive or continuous Client unable to stop cough Client uncomfortable May have fever	--YES→	CATEGORY III
Minor cough Client not appearing ill	--YES→	CATEGORY IV

COUGH
RESPIRATORY

Signs/Symptoms		Category
Croup cough with inspiratory and expiratory stridor Drooling	--YES→	CATEGORY I
Croup cough Not in acute distress	--YES→	CATEGORY II

CROUP-TYPE COUGH
RESPIRATORY

18

Signs/Symptoms

Category

Client showing active signs of
hemoptysis or history of
respiratory or cardiac disease
with hemoptysis

--YES→

CATEGORY I

Client history of coughing up
blood—small amount of thready
or pink tinged mucous
No previous history cardiac or
respiratory disease
Client does not appear ill

--YES→

CATEGORY III

HEMOPTYSIS
RESPIRATORY

18

Signs/Symptoms	Category
Hyperventilation symptoms currently active despite first aid	--YES→ CATEGORY II
Client presented with hyperventilation symptoms, but now shows no symptoms -or- Symptoms improved with first aid	--YES→ CATEGORY III

HYPERVENTILATION
RESPIRATORY

18

305

Signs/Symptoms

Client history of inhalation injury
Now showing signs of hypoxia, or
other distress

--YES→

Category

CATEGORY I

Client has history of inhalation injury
Currently showing no signs of injury

--YES→

CATEGORY III

INHALATION INJURY
RESPIRATORY

POSSIBLE FOREIGN BODY ASPIRATION
RESPIRATORY

Signs/Symptoms		Category
Breathing difficulty Cyanosis Decreased or absent breath sounds Continuous coughing Air hunger	--YES→	CATEGORY I
Periodic coughing No distress noted	--YES→	CATEGORY II
No noted respiratory distress No cough Client appears well	--YES→	CATEGORY IV

18

Signs/Symptoms	X-Ray/Lab		Category
Complaints of rib pain and shortness of breath following trauma			CATEGORY I
Complaints of rib pain following injury No complaints of shortness of breath	Rib x-ray	--YES→	CATEGORY III
Complaints of pinpoint rib pain with inspiration No history of injury		--YES→	CATEGORY IV

RIB PAIN
RESPIRATORY

Signs/Symptoms			Category
Client in respiratory distress	-or-	--YES→	CATEGORY I
History of cardiac problem / Now having shortness of breath or tachypnea, tachycardia, high blood pressure			
Complaints of shortness of breath / History of asthma, or other chronic breathing problems		--YES→	CATEGORY II
Client reports history of shortness of breath with exertion	-or-	--YES→	CATEGORY III
Client reports unable to get enough air because of pain with deep inspiration			

SHORTNESS OF BREATH RESPIRATORY

18

Signs/Symptoms

Client with tracheostomy
Tube coughed up
Client in respiratory distress

-or-

Client having problems with
tracheostomy but no acute
distress

Client with tracheostomy
Needs suctioning
Client having breathing difficulty

--YES→

--YES→

Category

CATEGORY I

CATEGORY II

**TRACHEOSTOMY
RESPIRATORY**

Signs/Symptoms

Client is having breathing difficulty
Wheeze, retracting
Decreased air movement
Nasal flare
Cyanosis or air hunger
Continuous cough

--YES→

Category

CATEGORY I

-or-

Possible sudden foreign body
aspiration
Not in acute distress

--YES→

CATEGORY II

All other wheezing
Known asthma

WHEEZE
RESPIRATORY

18

Category I	Category II	Category III	Category IV
Foreign body aspiration Breathing difficulty Hypoxia	Foreign body aspiration No distress	Cough Unable to stop Client uncomfortable and ill appearing	Foreign body aspiration—no cough Client appears well
Wheeze Client having breathing difficulty Respiratory distress	Known asthmatic—current wheeze No respiratory distress	Complaints of chest pain with breathing No cardiac history	Minor cough Client not appearing ill
Cough—continuous Client exhausted or in respiratory distress	Wheeze Possible foreign body aspiration		Mild congestion Client does not appear ill
Cough—client in distress History of cardiac or respiratory disease	Cough Possible foreign body aspiration	Hyperventilation Improving	Client reports unable to get enough air because of pain with deep inspiration
Breathing difficulty Chest pain May or may not have cardiac history	Infant: breathing difficulty Mild nasal flare Child irritable	Congested, ill Client fever over 101°	Congested Fever under 101°
Breathing difficulty Client irritable and ill appearing	Short of breath History of asthma or chronic breathing problems	Complaints of rib pain following injury No complaints of shortness of breath	Stuffy or runny nose
	Hyperventilation—current	Inhalation injury Showing no current problem	Complaints of rib pain with inspiration No history of injury
Short of breath Client in respiratory distress	Croup cough No acute distress	Client history of coughing up pink tinged mucous (no cardiac or respiratory disease)	Minor chest trauma Bruising may be present but no specific rib or breathing difficulties

History of cardiac problem
Now with symptoms

Infant
Cold, congestion
Mild nasal flaring
See-saw breathing

Croup cough
Client in distress

Breathing difficulties
associated with cold or
congestion

Chronic breathing problem
Now congested because
of cold
Client having difficulty
with tracheostomy
In no acute distress

Congested, irritable
Hypoxic client

Client with tracheostomy
Now in respiratory distress

Complaints of rib pain and
difficulty breathing (following
trauma)

Blunt chest injury and/
or rib pain
No respiratory distress

Client having active hemoptysis or
Now showing hypoxia or other
problems

Client having active hemopotysis or
history of cardiac or respiratory
disease with hemoptysis

Penetrating or blunt chest trauma
Client now showing signs of
respiratory distress

OVERVIEW
RESPIRATORY

18

MAJOR SYSTEM: TOXIC SUBSTANCES

Subjective and Objective Data

Contact Poisons

Medication Reaction

Toxic Bites and Stings

Flow Sheets

Contact Poisons

Medication Reaction

Toxic Bites and Stings

TOXIC SUBSTANCES

19

Subjective Assessment

1. Describe contact agent.

2. Length of time since contact.

3. First aid measures applied or home treatment methods since problem onset.

4. History of previous incident(s)—describe.

5. Description of symptoms now and progression of symptoms since contact.

6. Concurrent medical problems.

7. History of allergies.

Objective Assessment

1. Observation of affected area.

2. General observation of client health or distress.

SUBJECTIVE AND OBJECTIVE DATA—CONTACT POISONS TOXIC SUBSTANCES

Signs/Symptoms			Category
Accidental burn by caustic acid or alkali No first aid treatment <u>Client in distress</u>		--YES→	CATEGORY I
Accidental burn by caustic acid or alkali to face, eyes, mouth <u>First aid applied</u>	-or-	--YES→	CATEGORY II
	Contact with environmental substance Large body surface area covered or face and neck affected <u>Client feels ill</u>		
	-or-		
	Contact with environmental substance Allergic symptoms becoming worse <u>Client feels ill</u>		
Accidental burn by caustic acid or alkali First aid treatment applied No progression of injury <u>Client in no distress</u>		--YES→	CATEGORY III
Contact with environmental substance Minor allergic symptoms over local area Client uncomfortable but <u>in no distress</u>		--YES→	CATEGORY IV

CONTACT POISONS
TOXIC SUBSTANCES

19

317

Subjective Assessment

1. Type of drug currently being taken—describe how long medication has been used, what route, time of last dose, amount of dosage.

2. Previous history of drug reaction—this drug or others? Allergies in general?

3. Concurrent medical problems.

4. Other drugs currently being used.

5. Describe onset of problem—course of problem since onset.

6. Home treatment methods tried since onset of medication reaction.

7. Contact with contagious diseases or contact dermatitis in past two weeks.

8. Describe symptoms—respiratory system, G.I. system (nausea, vomiting, diarrhea, and pain or cramps), integumentary system (rash or itching).

Objective Assessment

1. General observation—appear ill?
   Integumentary (rash, hives, lesions, erythema)
   Respiratory (congestion, wheezing, shortness of breath, respiratory depression)
   Neurological status (level of consciousness, orientation)
   Cardiovascular (hypotension)

SUBJECTIVE AND OBJECTIVE DATA—MEDICATION REACTION TOXIC SUBSTANCES

Signs/Symptoms		Category
Systemic allergic response Client in respiratory or circulatory distress	--YES→	CATEGORY I
Systemic allergic response Severe G.I. response—vomiting, diarrhea or severe integumentary response—rash, hives No respiratory or circulatory symptoms	--YES→	CATEGORY II
Minor itching, rash or hives Allergic response Client uncomfortable but not ill	--YES→	CATEGORY III
Systemic response Minor G.I. symptoms only	--YES→	CATEGORY IV

MEDICATION REACTION TOXIC SUBSTANCES

19

Subjective Assessment

1. Describe type of bite or sting.

2. Length of time since bite/sting.

3. First aid measures applied.

4. Describe client reaction within first 10 minutes.

5. History of previous incident(s). Describe reaction at that time.

6. Concurrent medical problems.

7. History of allergies.

8. Description of how client is feeling now: respiratory system, G.I. system (nausea, vomiting, diarrhea, abdominal pain or cramps?).

Objective Assessment

1. Observation of bite/sting area—note general appearance, edema, erythema, number of bites or lesions.

2. Status of extremity distal to bite/sting.

3. General observation—appear ill?
   Respiratory (congestion, wheezing, shortness of breath, respiratory depression)
   Neurological status (level of consciousness, orientation)
   Cardiovascular (hypotension)

4. Assess for numbness, tingling, paresthesia of extremity or mouth.

SUBJECTIVE AND OBJECTIVE DATA—TOXIC BITES AND STINGS TOXIC SUBSTANCES

Signs/Symptoms		Category
History of bite/sting Client in respiratory distress; hypotension; neurological signs; ill appearing	-or-	--YES→ CATEGORY I
History of bite/sting Known poisonous substance No treatment or delayed treatment since injury Client in danger		
History of bite/sting Severe local reaction: pain, itching or tissue destruction No signs of systemic reaction		--YES→ CATEGORY II
History of bite/sting Minor local reaction No systemic reaction Local discomfort only		--YES→ CATEGORY IV

TOXIC BITES AND STINGS
TOXIC SUBSTANCES

19

Category I	Category II	Category III	Category IV
History of bite/sting Client in respiratory distress Hypotension; neurological signs ill appearing	History of bite/sting Severe local reaction Pain, itching or tissue destruction No signs of systemic reaction	Accidental burn by caustic acid or alkali First aid treatment applied No progression of injury Client in no distress	History of bite/sting Minor local reaction No systemic reaction Local discomfort only
History bite/sting; known poisonous substance No treatment or delayed treatment since injury Client in danger	Accidental burn by caustic acid or alkali to face, eyes, mouth First aid applied	Minor itching rash or hives Allergic response to medication Client uncomfortable but not ill	Contact with environmental substance Minor allergic symptoms over local area Client uncomfortable but in no distress
Accidental burn by caustic acid or alkali No first aid treatment Client in distress	Contact with environmental substance Large body surface area covered or face and neck affected Client feels ill		Systemic response to medication Minor G.I. symptoms only
Systemic allergic response to medication Client in respiratory or circulatory distress	Contact with environmental substance Allergic symptoms becoming worse Client feels ill		

OVERVIEW
TOXIC SUBSTANCES

Category I	Category II	Category III	Category IV
Systemic allergic response to medication Severe G.I. response—vomiting, diarrhea, or severe integumentary response—rash, hives No respiratory or circulatory symptoms			